THE EDUCATOR'S GUIDE
TO AIDS:
☐ *Law*
☐ *Medicine and*
☐ *Policy*

By Barbara Jean Harty-Golder

The Higher Education Administration Series
Edited by Donald D. Gehring and D. Parker Young

COLLEGE ADMINISTRATION PUBLICATIONS, INC.

© 1990, College Administration Publications, Inc.,
All rights reserved. Published 1990
Printed in the United States of America
94 93 92 91 90   5 4 3 2 1

Library of Congress Cataloging-in-Publication Data
Harty-Golder, Barbara Jean, 1951-
    The educators guide to AIDS: law, medicine and policy   /   by
Barbara Jean Harty-Golder.
        p.   cm.—(Higher education administration series)
    ISBN 0-912557-12-5 : $12.95
    1. AIDS (Disease)   2. AIDS (Disease)—Law and legislation—United
States   3. School management and organization—United States
I. Title.   II. Series.
    [DNLM: 1. Acquired Immunodeficiency Syndrome—legislation.
2. Attitude to Health.   3. Confidentiality—legislation.
4. Prejudice.   WD 308 H337e]
RA644.A25H38   1990
362.1'9697'9200973—dc20
DNLM/DLC
for Library of Congress   89-25250
                                                                 CIP

This publication is designed to provide accurate and authoritative information in regard to the subject matter covered. It is sold with the
understanding that the publisher is not engaged in rendering legal, ac-
counting or other professional service. If legal advice or other expert
assistance is required, the services of a competent professional person
should be sought.

*—from a Declaration of Principles jointly adopted by a committee of the American
Bar Association and a committee of publishers.*

To David, Reid and David

Table of Contents

Foreword

Without exception, every school administrator in the coming years will be faced with the problem of dealing with AIDS in educational institutions. The problems presented are not limited to determining the propriety and necessity of enrolling infected students, or of insuring the safety of the school environment. Administration officials will be faced with questions of confidentiality of medical information. They will be called on to determine when and whether classroom situations are placed at risk by HIV infected students, and whether and when the classroom environment becomes a risk to the student. Regulation of special programs, accommodation of the special needs of students suffering from symptomatic disease and the education of students and their parents about the reality of the disease AIDS have already become important issues at all levels of education.

A few short years ago, few questions concerning the impact of AIDS on education had concrete answers. Law scholars were uncertain whether this disease would be treated as a public health issue alone, or whether the overlay of civil rights issues would ultimately determine the direction in which courts and legislators would resolve issues of attendance, confidentiality and testing. In a relatively short time, by case law and legislative pronouncements, many of the fundamental issues regarding the proper treatment of infected individuals have been resolved. Out of a background of confusions, some clear directions and imperatives have emerged. Great public debate still flourishes on the relative wisdom and propriety of some of these decisions, but they have finally been clearly made. Administrators at all levels are faced with the necessity of bringing school policies in line with stringent new requirements of law. Failure to do so, whether by ignorance or design, is costly, as more and more cases claiming discrimination, or breach of confidentiality on the basis of HIV infection reach the courts and are resolved in favor of the plaintiff.

In order to formulate proper policy, an administrator must first have accurate knowledge of the biology of HIV infection and be conversant with the principles of public health, discrimination and tort law which are the foundation of social policy regarding AIDS. Nowhere in the law is a detailed knowledge of science and law more important than in the area of formulating effective and legally permissible policies for dealing with AIDS in the educational environment. Blanket policies, particularly if they serve to discriminate against HIV infected individuals, have little real utility and are suspect under law. Each HIV infected student in each school and college environment presents some unique features, and these must be individually evaluated to insure proper attention to the concerns of all parties involved.

It is the purpose of this monograph to provide appropriate background information about the science and the law concerning AIDS. It is science and law which mold the analysis and thought which are necessary for designing policies which are not only currently appropriate, but capable of the flexibility to meet future issues as well. The final chapters will deal with common problems encountered in educational environments and provide models for managing environmental problems, accommodating infected students, and testing and screening programs. Dealing with AIDS requires sufficient understanding of underlying social policy to know when blanket policies are inappropriate, and how particular issues must be individually addressed to keep within the spirit and the letter of the law as shaped by the dictates of scientific understanding.

About the Author

BARBARA JEAN HARTY-GOLDER earned her M.D. with honors from the University of Florida College of Medicine in 1977. She has served as a hospital based pathologist specializing in hematopathology and oncologic pathology, as an assistant professor of Pathology at Oregon Health Sciences University and as an associate medical examiner specializing in forensic medicine. Dr. Harty-Golder received her J.D. magna cum laude from Stetson University College of Law in 1988, where she was the recipient of the Walter Mann Award. Dr. Harty-Golder was admitted to the Florida Bar in 1988. She is a member of the Tort and Insurance Practice, Anti-Trust, Health Law, and Science and Technology sections of the American Bar Association.

Dr. Harty-Golder has lectured and taught in the area of AIDS Law since 1985. She has recently co-authored a chapter on AIDS and Employment Law *Labour and Employment Law in Florida: Law, Policy and Practice* (Vol. II). Published by Stetson University College of Law (due out in early 1990). Her other areas of interest are Death and Dying Law and Health Care Risk Management.

Introduction

> The "Red Death" had long devastated the country. No pestilence had ever been so fatal, or so hideous. Blood was its Avatar and its seal—the redness and horror of blood. There were sharp pains and sudden dizziness, and the profuse bleeding at the pores, with dissolution. The scarlet stains upon the body and especially upon the face of the victim were the pest-ban which shut him out from the aid and from the sympathy of his fellow man.
>
> —Edgar Allen Poe
> "The Masque of the Red Death"

Poe's fable presents some disturbing similarities to the progression of the AIDS epidemic in modern America. His protagonist, Prince Prospero, in an attempt to flee the plague abroad in the countryside, shuts himself and his courtiers apart from the world, in a walled city; and then celebrates secure in his belief that he is at last free from the dreaded disease. Ultimately, of course, his plan fails; the Red Death is discovered among the revelers themselves.

Like the mythical sufferers of the Red Death, people with AIDS all too often find themselves shut off from the aid, sympathy and society of others. The public sees AIDS as "somebody else's" disease. In attempts to avoid the sick in an effort to avoid the disease, fearful communities have shunned infected school children, picketed schoolhouses, issued death threats and burned homes. "Safe sex" clubs whose members are regularly tested for infection have sprung up in a chilling mockery of Prospero's court, and equally destined to failure.

All too often, AIDS is the story of young people dying suddenly, unexpectedly and alone. The AIDS patient faces a course of increasing debility and disfigurement as the disease takes its inexorable toll. Economic impoverishment is not uncommon because of large medical bills and jobs lost either to the effects of the disease or the effects of prejudice. Family and friends, fearful of infection and reluctant to accept the lifestyle which may have contributed to it, often abandon the infected individual. Among members of high risk groups, "grief overload" is common, as they watch dozens of friends die painful, protracted deaths.

The tragedy of AIDS is only compounded by public fear and unwillingness to accept AIDS for what it is: an infectious disease, communicated primarily by sexual activity and drug use, presenting no risk of transmission from truly casual contact. AIDS is no longer a disease of the homosexual community, but of mainstream, heterosexual America. The legitimate precautionary measures necessary to prevent spread of the disease are simple and behavioral: avoiding promiscuous sex and eliminating contact with blood and body fluids which might be contaminated. Since the vast majority of human interaction involves neither of these activities, AIDS patients can, with few exceptions, remain a functioning part of society while posing no real risk to the people around them. All that remains is for the rest of society to accept people with AIDS and let them get on with the rest of their lives.

The legal framework exists to help insure the place of AIDS patients in society. Our challenge now must be to develop attitudes of caring, understanding and support. Any policy which fails to affirm the dignity and relieve the personal suffering of people with AIDS fails also to recognize that the AIDS epidemic touches us all. Prospero and his courtiers paid a heavy price for the same mistake:

> And now was acknowledged the presence of the Red Death. He had come like a thief in the night. And one by one dropped the revelers in the blood-bedewed halls of their revels . . . And Darkness and Decay and the Red Death held illimitable dominion over all.

Without exception, every institutional administrator in the coming years will be faced with the problem of dealing with AIDS in the nation's schools and colleges. The problems presented are not limited to determining the propriety and necessity of enrolling infected students, or of insuring the safety of the educational environment. Administrative officials will be faced with questions of confidentiality of medical information. They will be called on to determine when and whether classroom situations are placed at risk by HIV infected students, and whether and when the classroom environment becomes a risk to the student. Regulation of special programs, accommodation of the special needs of students suffering from symptomatic disease and the education of students and their parents about the reality of the disease AIDS have already become important issues at all levels of education.

A few short years ago, few questions concerning the impact of AIDS on education had concrete answers. Law scholars were uncertain whether this disease would be treated as a public health issue alone, or whether the overlay of civil rights issues would ultimately determine the direction in which courts and legislators would resolve issues of attendance, confidentiality and testing. In a relatively short time, by case law and legislative pronouncements, many of the fundamental issues regarding the proper treatment of infected individuals have been resolved. Out of a background of confusions, some clear directions and imperatives have emerged. Great public debate still flourishes on the relative wisdom and propriety of some of these decisions, but they have finally been clearly made. Administrators at all levels are faced with the necessity of bringing institution policies in line with stringent new requirements of law. Failure to do so, whether by ignorance or design, is costly, as more and more cases claiming discrimination, or breach of confidentiality on the basis of HIV infection reach the courts and are resolved in favor of the plaintiff.

In order to formulate proper policy, an administrator must first have accurate knowledge of the biology of HIV infection and be conversant with the principles of public health, discrimination and tort law which are the foundation of social policy regarding AIDS. Nowhere in the law is a detailed knowledge of science and law more important than in the area of formulating effective and legally permissible policies for dealing with AIDS in the school environment. Blanket policies, particularly if they serve to discriminate against HIV infected individuals, have little real utility and are suspect under law. Each HIV infected student in each school or college environment presents some unique features, and these must be individually evaluated to insure proper attention to the concerns of all parties involved.

It is the purpose of this monograph to provide appropriate background information about the science and the law concerning AIDS. It is science and law which mold the analysis and thought which are necessary for designing policies which are not only currently appropriate, but capable of the flexibility to meet future issues as well. The final chapters of this book will deal with common problems encountered in educational environments and provide models for managing environmental problems, accommodating infected students, and testing and screening programs. Dealing with AIDS requires sufficient understanding of underlying social policy to know when blanket policies are inappropriate, and how particular issues must be individually addressed to keep within the spirit and the letter of the law as shaped by the dictates of scientific understanding and social conscience.

Institutional administrators and policymakers have an opportunity to demonstrate to the public at-large how the problems presented by the AIDS epidemic can be handled with compassion, concern and intelligence, to protect the needs of all of us. As we are all touched by this disease, directly or indirectly, schools and colleges must play a central role in educating us that we can live safely with the specter of HIV infection and with infected people in our midst as long as we learn what is necessary for our protection and change our behaviors accordingly. Defusing the irrational public fear of AIDS can only begin by demonstrating commitment to scientifically sound and socially sensitive policies in our public institutions. There is no better place to begin than in the nation's educational institutions.

Chapter I

Epidemiological Background
Of The AIDS Epidemic

Acquired Immune Deficiency Syndrome (AIDS) was first recognized in the United States in 1981, based on observations of Dr. Michael Gottlieb of the University of California at Los Angeles. Dr. Gottlieb followed a series of young homosexual men who were being treated for unusual infections which do not ordinarily affect individuals with healthy immune systems. The fact that these patients had none of the usual factors, such as immune deficiency present from birth, or treatment with steroids or anti-cancer drugs known to produce immune defects which are responsible for immune compromise, made their cases both noteworthy and worrisome. By 1982, other researchers had noted the association of immune compromise, unusual cancers and infections in young, homosexual men, and the name "acquired immune deficiency syndrome (AIDS)" was ultimately coined to describe this new disease. Although the beginning of the AIDS epidemic is generally taken to be the mid to late 1970's, recent studies show that sporadic cases were present in the United States even prior to that time.

Subsequently, a related condition, designated AIDS Related Complex (ARC) was also coined to describe individuals who demonstrated some immune deficiency and mild symptoms, but who lacked the characteristic cancers and infections associated with cases of AIDS. Suspicion was high that AIDS was an infectious disease and by 1984, the infectious agent had been independently identified by researchers in France and the U.S. The causative agent of AIDS and ARC is a virus which was independently named Human T-Lymphotrophic Virus III (HTLV-III), Lymphadenopathy Associated Virus (LAV), and Human Immunodeficiency Virus (HIV). For purposes of simplicity, the infectious agent of AIDS will be designated HIV throughout this monograph.

1

SPECTRUM OF HIV INFECTIONS

HIV infection may take many forms which blend into one another in a spectrum ranging from apparent good health with no symptoms to the full-blown immune compromise and debility which characterizes AIDS. Initially, infection with HIV is silent and produces virtually no symptoms, although a transient, flu-like or encephalitis-like illness may occur at the time of initial infection. For an extended period, the only indication of infection is the presence of antibody to HIV in the blood or the presence of the virus itself in blood samples. The majority of HIV infections fall into this category of latent or silent infection. Despite the lack of symptoms, individuals infected with HIV are capable of transmitting the infection. Most cases of transmission probably occur out of this group.

The next step in the progression of the disease is AIDS-Related Complex (ARC), characterized by the development of physical symptoms, such as weight loss, enlargement of lymph nodes and fatigue, with concurrent abnormalities in the immune system which can be measured by laboratory tests. (Table I) This is also characterized by

TABLE I

Criteria for Diagnosis of AIDS Related Complex (ARC)

Criteria	Findings
Clinical:	• fever for more than three months • weight loss greater than 10% of body weight • enlargement of lymph nodes longer than three months • diarrhea • fatigue • night sweats
Laboratory:	• decreased T-helper cells • decreased ratio of T-helper to T-suppressor cells • increased serum globulins • inability to respond to immune stimuli (anergy) • decreased ability of lymphocytes to respond to mitogens

active proliferation of the virus within the infected lymphocytes. Current estimates are that approximately 40% of HIV infected individuals will develop ARC within two years of infection.

Finally, full-blown AIDS may develop as a result of HIV infection. A diagnosis of AIDS is confirmed by confirming the presence of particular clinical manifestations which are determined by the Centers for Disease Control (CDC) as diagnostic of full-blown AIDS. The clinical criteria for designation of AIDS have expanded since the disease was initially identified·as studies have revealed the multitude of forms this infection may take once it becomes symptomatic. As now defined,

2

AIDS is clinically characterized by severe immune deficiency, resulting in unusual infections and the occurrence of various, otherwise uncommon cancers. (Table II) AIDS results in increased destruction of the

TABLE II

Criteria for Diagnosis of AIDS

Criteria	Diagnosis
Infections:	• Protozoal and helminthic infections: *Pneumocystis carinii pneumonia* (PCP), toxoplasmosis, cryptosporidiosis, strongyloidiasis, isosporiasis • Fungal infections: thrush (Candida infection of the mouth), deep (lung, bronchial or other tissue) infection with Candida, cryptococcosis • Infections with atypical variants of tuberculosis, including *Mycobacterium kansasii* and *M. avium-interacellulare.* • Widespread or chronic viral infections: Herpes simplex, Cytomegalovirus • Progressive multifocal leucoencephalopathy
Malignancies:	• Kaposi's sarcoma, in young men (less than sixty years) lymphoma limited to the brain lymphoma associated with infections (above) • aggressive non-Hosgkin's lymphoma
Other:	• chronic lymphoid interstitial pneumonitis (in children under thirteen • changes in mental status (dementia)

cells of the immune system, and as this change progresses, the disease becomes progressively worse. AIDS patients manifest a variety of illnesses such as recurrent pneumonia, parasitic infections of the bowel, encephalitis and neurological changes which range from forgetfulness to psychosis. AIDS, once developed, is uniformly fatal, usually within a year of diagnosis. There is some evidence that AIDS is more rapidly progressive in women and drug users than in homosexual men with no history of drug use. No conclusive explanation has yet been found for this discrepancy, but it may relate to the fact that many female AIDS patients are also drug abusers (54%), and drug abusers, because of poor health, nutrition and immune deficiency, as a result of their habit may consequently suffer more drastically from the effects of infection, once manifest.

Initial studies indicated that only about 10% of HIV infected individuals would eventually develop AIDS. More recent data indicate that percentage to be substantially higher. Current figures are 50%. Other, more ominous projections range in excess of 75%. Even more worrisome is the fact that, so far, the percentage of individuals developing AIDS increases with increasing time, showing no signs of plateau. Because HIV infection is life-long, this raises the possibility that, ultimately, nearly all patients who are infected may ultimately develop symptomatic disease, given sufficient time. Because our estimates of the number of HIV infected individuals who are asymptomatic are only approximate, the actual percentage of individuals who go on to develop symptomatic disease and die, is uncertain. The currently accepted figure of 50% is certainly a minimum estimate.

The latent period between initial infection and the development of the clinical symptoms of AIDS or ARC can be quite long, averaging from five to ten years. Thus, it is not possible to predict if, when, or in what way infection will ultimately become symptomatic in any particular individual.

The CDC has further subdivided the spectrum of HIV infection into five stages. Stages I and II correspond to asymptomatic infection, Stage III corresponds roughly to ARC, and Stages IV and V represent full-blown AIDS. A separate classification system exists to categorize infection in children, who have different clinical responses to HIV infection. This confusion of classification symptoms, and the subjectivity of evaluation, especially of ARC, sometimes makes it difficult to understand precisely what is meant by the terms AIDS and ARC, and how they interrelate. The most productive way in which to view HIV infection is as a spectrum, ranging from silent infection to unequivocal AIDS, with ARC a condition somewhere in between. Clinical manifestations shade from one condition to another, often without clearcut distinction.

Although it appears that the infectivity of an individual waxes and wanes throughout the course of the disease, it cannot be correlated to antibody level, stage of disease, or other identifiable factors. Thus, any individual demonstrating HIV in the blood or anti-HIV antibody must be considered continuously and permanently capable of transmitting infection to others. It is further important to recognize that anyone demonstrating antibody to HIV, confirmed by appropriate tests, has not only been exposed to HIV, but is also infected, regardless of the clinical symptoms he does or does not demonstrate.

TRANSMISSION OF HIV INFECTION

HIV infection is transmitted by contact of infected blood or body fluids from an infected individual to an uninfected person. Most commonly, this occurs during sexual intercourse; hence, HIV infection may be legitimately designated, at least in part, a venereal disease. Male and female genital secretions contain large numbers of virus particles. The presence of cuts, tears or abrasions on the mucous membranes increase the likelihood of infection. Consequently, anal sex, with its high incidence of tissue injury, is more likely to transmit HIV than vaginal intercourse, although vaginal intercourse is perfectly effective in transmission of infection. Oral sex may also result in infection, since passage of the virus may occur through any mucous membrane.

Direct bloodstream contact with contaminated blood may also transmit HIV infection. Transfusion of infected blood products has been largely controlled in the United States because of screening procedures, but is still common in underdeveloped nations which cannot afford the expense of screening the blood supply. Transmission by shared needle use among addicts has also become a significant means of spread of the disease.

Of increasing concern is the population of children who acquire the infection across the placenta or from contaminated breast milk. Because HIV infection can remain silent for many years, the first evidence a woman has that she is infected with the virus may be the birth of a child with AIDS.

Thus, the main routes of HIV infection are sexual intercourse, by far the predominant route; drug abuse, transfusion of contaminated blood and intrauterine infection. However, the fact that a constant 1-3% of cases cannot be associated with any known risk factors, and the occasional reports of infection acquired in other ways by contact with infected blood or body fluids, emphasizes that any contact with infected blood or body fluids poses some risk. The CDC reported three cases of HIV infection acquired when health care workers with broken skin came in contact with infected blood, a mode of transmission previously not recognized. Infection by accidental needle stick has also been reported, although the rate of infection after accidental needlestick exposure is extremely low, less than 1%. An infected mother who acquired infection after the birth of her child subsequently passed the infection through breast milk. A single case of HIV infection transmitted to the caregiver of an infant with severe, continuous, bloody diarrhea has been reported, as has one transmission between siblings, apparently by biting. These routes of transmission so far represent only an extremely small fraction of HIV infections. Further, extensive studies of non-sexual household contacts of AIDS patients has demonstrated no increased risk of acquiring infection, even among those assisting in home administration of blood products to hemophiliacs who run an increased risk of accidental needlestick. The risk of acquiring postnatal infection by activities other than intercourse, drug abuse or receipt of infected blood products is quite remote, although not nonexistent.

RISK GROUPS AND AIDS

Recognition of AIDS as an infectious disease prompted early recognition and definition of groups at particular risk for acquiring the disease. Initially, the defined risk groups were limited to homosexual males, Haitians and drug abusers. We now know that this emphasis on risk groups rather than risky behavior is inappropriate. Current understanding indicates that risk is related to personal habits and behavior, not identity with any particular social or ethnic group.

Individuals who are sexually promiscuous, abuse drugs, or who had blood transfusions prior to the implementation of effective screening programs, are those at risk of acquiring the disease, regardless of the demographic group in which they fall.

Because HIV infection may be spread venereally, any sexually active person is at risk to acquire the disease once the infection is present among his or her sexual contacts. HIV infection first appeared in America among homosexual males. Initially, nearly all cases of AIDS were found among homosexual males, and, although initially unrecognized, cases among drug abusers and infants of drug abusers also surfaced early. AIDS in America remains predominantly a disease of homosexual males, but cases among heterosexuals are increasing rapidly and can be expected to continue to increase as HIV infection becomes more disseminated in the heterosexual population. Heterosexual AIDS will be a significant problem in the coming decades.

Because HIV infection may be transmitted by contaminated blood, any activity which transfers blood from one individual to another constitutes a risk. Intravenous drug abusers compose a large, at-risk population: 50% of drug abusers tested in New York City were infected with HIV. Although a number of ethnic groups are disproportionately represented among drug abusers, notably blacks and Hispanics in some major metropolitan centers, the risk of acquiring HIV infection stems from personal habits, not ethnic origin.

Until 1984, there was no specific screening test capable of identifying infected units of blood, and a number of cases of HIV infection resulted from transfusion of infected blood and blood products prior to 1985. Transfusion-related AIDS occurs in all ages, and is related only to receiving contaminated blood products. It has been reported in premature infants requiring transfusion, as well as adult patients undergoing surgery requiring transfusion. HIV infection is extremely common among hemophiliacs, who require large amounts of commercially obtained pooled clotting factors for control of their disease. Of all AIDS cases reported, 1% occur in hemophiliacs, but 75% of hemophiliacs who required clotting factors prior to 1985 are infected with HIV.

Since the institution of screening procedures, cases of transfusion related HIV infection have been almost eliminated. Because there is a biological lag time between infection and development of the antibody identified by the screening test, occasional cases of transfusion related infection are still reported. HIV infection resulting from organ transplantation has also occurred, as has infection from artificial insemination, because seminal fluid contains large amounts of virus particles.

Interestingly, the identification of the risk of hematogenous transmission of HIV infection to the public initially resulted in a reluctance to donate blood. Since HIV infection is associated with receiving, rather than donating, infected blood, blood donation is an activity completely without risk for acquiring the disease.

Relatively little is known about the individual factors which predispose to, or might protect from, HIV infection. It has become clear, for example, that the clinical course of AIDS varies among individuals. Some are likely to develop Kaposi's sarcoma, a malignant tumor of blood vessels. Others are more likely to develop *Pneumocystis carinii pneumonia* (PCP), a parasitic infection of the lung. Further, which of these two diseases is the primary manifestation of the disease relates to the ultimate survival, and as increasing numbers of patients receive updated therapy, some longer term survivors have emerged. Other studies demonstrate that some known sexual contacts of HIV infected individuals remain uninfected. These data indicate that there may be host factors which affect the rate of infection or the course of the disease but there has been no convincing explanation for these phenomena. It is thought that underlying immune stress or compromise might predispose to infection and to the likelihood of developing of symptomatic disease, as might repeated exposure to the virus and the concentration of virus in contaminated fluids.

WORLDWIDE AIDS

Africa appears to have been the site in which HIV infection originated, and the most extensive endemic infection of populations occurs there. It is referred to as "slim" because of the emaciation the later stages of the disease produces in its victims.

HIV infection in Africa is transmitted predominantly by heterosexual contact, and the number of infected males and females is equal. Another significant risk factor in the epidemiology of African AIDS is the use of common needles for injection, ritual scarification, and the significant contamination of the blood supply because of the high rate of infection among the general population. The fact that HIV infection in Africa is largely a heterosexual disease confirms that the initial confinement of AIDS to the homosexual population in the United States was an epidemiological fluke, reflecting social and personal habits rather than any inherent susceptibility to the disease. It further underscores that current articles in the lay press suggesting that the risk for heterosexual transmission of HIV infection is low are erroneous. It cannot be over emphasized. Once HIV infection is present among an individual's sexual contacts, however acquired, the risk of transmission by homosexual or heterosexual intercourse is substantial.

Examination of the population in endemic areas has produced some interesting information about HIV infection. Some subpopulations of Africa exhibit antibodies to a virus related to HIV, but not known to produce immune deficiency, which raises the hope that a vaccine to prevent HIV infection may be practical. And, although HIV has been reported isolated from mosquitoes, the epidemiology of the disease in the endemic areas of Africa excludes supporting a role for mosquito borne infection. Mosquito borne diseases are typically more prevalent in children than adults, as is the case for malaria, also endemic in the areas where AIDS is common. AIDS in those areas remains largely an adult disease, excluding cases of verifiable intrauterine transmission. Insect vectors do not appear to transmit HIV infection.

MAGNITUDE OF THE PROBLEM

Any discussion of statistics of the AIDS epidemic must take into account the fact that, because of the extremely long latency the virus may demonstrate, current disease patterns represent infections which resulted years before. Further, estimates of HIV infection among the general population are sketchy, since no screening data are available for the population at large. As of July 1987, the number of cases of symptomatic AIDS in the United States was over 42,000. Deaths from AIDS totaled 23,000. Estimates of asymptomatic infection range as high as 2 million overall. Among certain groups with common risk factors, the percentage of individuals is very high: approximately 75% of hemophiliacs, 50% of drug users in major metropolitan areas, 75% of the homosexual community in San Francisco, 20% of prostitutes in Miami. Even more ominous are recent preliminary findings that approximately 3% of entering college students demonstrated antibody to HIV.

Once ARC or AIDS is diagnosed, the cost of individual care can run as high as $150,000. Some experts place the anticipated cost of caring for AIDS patients at $37 billion by the year 1990. The challenge of caring for an extremely ill, often uninsured and generally young population with a fatal disease which requires enormous amounts of expensive care will shape the course of American health care in the decades to come.

AIDS has begun to make inroads to the general population, reflecting once again that its early confinement to the homosexual population was an epidemiological coincidence. The number of heterosexually transmitted cases doubled between 1985 and 1986. Likewise, the number of cases of pediatric AIDS has increased rapidly, and currently represents in excess of 500 cases. Although homosexually transmitted HIV infection will continue to be a significant problem, it is expected that heterosexually transmitted infection will become increasingly more common in the next decade. AIDS is unequivocally a health problem of the general public and will continue to be so for the foreseeable future.

Chapter II

The Biology of HIV Infection

HIV is a retrovirus: a virus which contains RNA as its genetic material, and utilizes the cellular machinery of the host cell to make a copy of its own RNA into DNA for reproduction. This is accomplished by an enzyme, reverse transcriptase, which is contained within the virus particle itself. It also belongs to the subgroup of retroviruses called lentiviruses, which are viruses characteristically demonstrating long latent periods between infection and symptomatic disease.

HIV demonstrates a predilection for infecting cells of the immune system, predominantly lymphocytes, and the nervous system, which accounts for the predominance of immunologic and neurological abnormalities in those infected by the virus. This is a result of the affinity of the virus for a cell surface marker called T4 antigen (also known as CD4), present on the surface of cells of the immune system as well as those of the nervous system. HIV binds to the T4 protein, enters the cell and breaks up into its component parts.

Once the virus has entered the host cell, the enzyme, reverse transcriptase, produces a copy of DNA from the viral RNA. This DNA becomes incorporated into the host cell's genetic information and accounts for the persistence of infection by HIV, as well as its long latency. This latency can be interrupted, and the virus activated, by stimulation of the infected cell by other viruses or antigens. Activated virus uses the host cellular machinery to reproduce viral RNA and proteins, with new, completely formed virus particles ultimately budding from the cell surface.

Because stimulation is known to be partially responsible for activation of the virus within the cell, ultimately causing viral reproduction and death of host lymphocytes, it is thought that recurrent infections and exposure to high levels of antigens may play a role in accelerating symptomatic disease in infected individuals. For this reason,

HIV positive individuals are counseled to avoid activities which stress the immune system, and exposure to infections and antigenic proteins.

HIV is a highly variable virus, demonstrating frequent changes in the molecular composition of the viral coat. Because the development of an effective vaccine depends in large measure on a stable virus structure, the variability of HIV poses significant problems for the development of a protective vaccine, as does the fact that antibody produced by virus infected individuals is not protective. Studies have also demonstrated constant areas of the viral surface which may be amenable to vaccine production, but the development of a vaccine capable of eliciting a protective antibody in the recipient is years in the future. Nevertheless, the development of a commercially sound and medically safe vaccine capable of preventing infection would undoubtedly be the ideal way to contain the AIDS epidemic.

Despite its virulent nature, HIV is a fragile virus, incapable of prolonged exposure to environments outside the host cell. It is rapidly deactivated by drying as well as heat sterilization. Common household bleach is sufficient to inactivate HIV, and in dilute solution (1:10) is the recommended agent for disinfecting spills of blood or body fluids. Because of its fragility, HIV infection is not transmitted by contact with surfaces such as doorknobs, or toilet seats. The fragility of HIV outside the body accounts in part for the fact that casual contact is not a risk in the transmission of infection.

Chapter III

Laboratory Diagnosis of HIV Infection

RELATIONSHIP OF INFECTION TO ANTIBODY RESPONSE

As is typical of viral exposure, HIV infection results in the production of virus-specific antibody which is carried in the bloodstream. The presence of this virus-specific antibody is the basis of current laboratory tests for HIV infection. Although it is possible to isolate infective virus particles from the blood and tissues of HIV infected individuals, and thus confirm the presence of infection, such isolation techniques are too cumbersome and expensive to use for routine screening.

After initial infection by HIV, there is a lag period during which the individual is infected by virus and capable of transmitting disease but demonstrates no antibody. It was initially thought that the lag period would not exceed six months, but more recent data indicates that in some individuals, the production of antibody may be delayed for as long as one to two years after initial infection. A single negative antibody test, therefore, does not indicate freedom from infection. If, however, after a single exposure, no antibody is demonstrated after testing at intervals ranging from six weeks to two years, the individual is assumed to be free of infection.

A single exposure is sufficient to transmit infection, however, and each new exposure begins the potential lag period again. Continuing exposure, such as frequent sexual activity with multiple partners, or drug abuse, thus makes it impossible to exclude infection on the basis of a single, or even repeated, negative antibody test.

Antibody levels in HIV infection vary among patients, and may wax and wane in a single patient during the course of the disease. What relationship antibody levels have to the course of disease has not yet been determined. Except in the case of passively acquired antibody, like that in newborns, who may acquire antibody from their mother's bloodstream without actually being infected by the virus, the presence of confirmed antibody to HIV is indicative of infection. All individuals who demonstrate antibodies to HIV must also be considered infectious to others in the proper circumstances.

LABORATORY TESTS FOR ANTIBODIES TO HIV

It was soon recognized that, although individuals with HIV infection may demonstrate clinical and laboratory abnormalities indicating immune compromise, not all infected individuals will do so. Thus, it was of considerable clinical importance to develop an antibody test capable of screening out infected individuals whose infection was clinically silent. The test needed to be relatively simple, cost-effective, and sensitive enough to detect all cases of HIV infection.

It was from this background that antibody tests for HIV infection were developed. Currently, screening tests initially designed to identify infected blood donors are coupled with confirmatory tests when absolute documentation of HIV infection is necessary in an individual case.

Because screening of blood donors requires only that all potentially infected units be identified, the screening test used can, and does, have a relatively high rate of false positive results. The test is designed to detect even a small amount of antibody, but is consequently less specific for HIV infection. Thus, a certain percentage of individuals who test positive for antibody on the screening test are not actually infected with HIV. In screening blood donors, no further test is required: the positive unit is simply discarded since it is safer and more cost-effective to discard potentially usable units which test falsely positive for HIV infection than to undertake the expense of confirming the results.

However, in identifying and counseling individuals who are potentially infected with HIV, the rate of false positive results from a screening test is unacceptably high. Therefore, in evaluation of individual patients, confirmatory tests must be undertaken to determine which positive results on screening actually represent infection with HIV.

The screening test used most commonly in detection of HIV infection is an enzyme linked assay (ELISA). In screening donated blood, a positive reaction to the ELISA test results in discard of the affected unit of blood, even though the ELISA test has a very high false positive rate.

If an individual tests positive on a single ELISA screening test, it is very possible that the result does not represent infection by HIV. In a population known to have a low incidence of infection, the likelihood that a positive ELISA is indicative of infection is approximately 15%. In a population with a high prevalence of infection, the significance of a positive result is much higher, and may approach 90%. Performance of a second ELISA will eliminate some false positive results, but absolute and reliable confirmation requires the performance of a more specific test designed to detect only the antibodies which represent HIV infection. Diagnosis of HIV infection should never be made on the basis of positive ELISA tests alone.

The most common confirmatory test currently used is called the Western Blot test, which is a very specific test examining specific protein antibodies to individual viral components derived from disrupted viral particles. It is an expensive, difficult, subjective and time consuming test, but highly accurate for identification of HIV infection. A positive ELISA followed by a confirmatory Western Blot test is interpreted as indicative of HIV infection although very rarely, false positive results also occur with the Western Blot. Correlation of the levels of antibody "titre" in both tests with a good clinical history will significantly reduce the small error involved in confirmatory testing, and should reduce the number of false positive results to the smallest number humanly possible (Kaplan, 1986). New confirmatory tests utilizing recombinant viral proteins and objective endpoints for testing may replace the Western Blot as the confirmatory test of choice, and offer the possibility of further decreasing the incidence of indeterminate or false positive results. No laboratory test can ever be guaranteed absolutely free of erroneous results, however, and the tests designed to detect HIV infection are no exception.

Thus, programs offering testing for HIV antibody need to include counseling and professional interpretation of clinical and laboratory data, rather than just providing raw test results. Public health programs offering voluntary testing have adopted this approach, first screening patients with sequential ELISA tests, confirming positive results with a Western Blot, and providing counseling and interpretation before, during and following the testing procedures. Some state laws which control testing for HIV, mandate this procedure in any situation where HIV testing is done. It is also important to realize that the test procedures for detecting HIV infection are rather complicated, requiring considerable experience and rigorous quality control. An unfortunate side effect of the AIDS epidemic has been an expansion of unqualified laboratories offering testing for HIV infection without proper experience or safeguards, resulting in unacceptably high rates of false results as well as a proportion of false negative ones. Any testing program must affiliate only with the most cautious and technologically competent laboratory available. Local public health officers will generally be able to provide references to the most appropriate laboratories in the area. "At home" test kits, which are not legally available in some states, are unsuitable for any sort of HIV testing, and their use should be discouraged.

A small percentage of patients who are infected with HIV will not produce antibody, and some patients with full-blown AIDS lose the ability to produce antibody during the course of their disease. Thus, there exists a very small population of HIV infected individuals who will not test positive for antibody and represent false-negative results. Recently, researchers have announced a test for viral antigens present early in infection which precede the development of antibody, and which appear to be lost later on in the course of infection, which may provide another method for determining infection in antibody negative individuals early in the course of disease.

Infants born to mothers who are infected with HIV present a particular problem in diagnosis since they may acquire the specific antibody passively from the mother without being infected with the virus. Thus, the presence of HIV antibody in the newborn is not necessarily indicative of infection, unless it can be demonstrated by confirmatory testing that the antibody is not of maternal origin. This is generally accomplished by examining the subtype of antibody produced to determine whether it is of small enough molecular weight to have passed through the placental barrier. If not, the antibody must have been generated by the infant, and is indicative of infection. Isolation of the virus from the infant's blood can also be done to confirm infection.

ANCILLARY TESTS

In addition to antibody testing, it is possible to isolate virus from infected individuals. This procedure is particularly time consuming and expensive, and adds little to clinical information supplemented by the more standardized screening and confirmatory tests. Thus, it is generally used only in research settings and to identify infection in newborns, since isolation of virus from an individual is certain proof of infection.

Because many patients with HIV infection are also infected by other viruses (hepatitis B, cytomegalovirus), they will demonstrate antibodies to other viral agents as well. These antibodies were considered as surrogate tests for HIV infection prior to the development of HIV specific antibody techniques, but are of little clinical importance in the diagnosis of HIV infection since the evolution of HIV specific tests.

Clinical management of the patient with HIV infection, as well as research, may require specific examination of immune functions. Laboratory abnormalities in the numbers and types of lymphocytes, the levels of gamma globulin and clinical evidence of immune defi-

14

ciency such as inability to react to skins tests have all been documented in HIV infected patients, and are clinically useful in following the course of infection.

Chapter IV

Low Risk Behavior:
What Is Casual Contact?

The routes by which HIV infection is transmitted are now fairly well defined: acquiring infection requires contact with infected blood or body fluids. Because the virus is very fragile outside the body, it is not spread by the casual human contact which makes up most activity in workplaces and educational institutions. Thus, there is no medical basis for broad exclusionary policies preventing HIV infected individuals from participating in normal daily activities.

Despite this, a great public concern remains about the rare occasional transmission of HIV infection by routes other than sexual activity, needle sharing or receiving infected blood products. On the one hand, the public is constantly being reassured that HIV infection presents essentially no risk in the usual educational or workplace environment. On the other hand, the public is increasingly aware of the stringent infection control measures being implemented by the health profession in its daily contact with patients. It becomes difficult for parents of school aged children, for example, to understand why they should not be concerned with the possibility that their child will be exposed to HIV infection because of a playmate's bloody nose when it is now routine for health care workers to don gloves, and occasionally masks and gowns, before caring for patients. Such a perceived double standard has been cited as a factor in the controversy which erupted in Arcadia, Florida, over the enrollment of three HIV infected children in public schools. A local physician, noting that a large part of the local population is employed either at a nearby state prison or the local state hospital where stringent infection control procedures are the rule, summed up the situation thus:

> When parents are told one thing at the place they work about wearing gloves, masks, goggles to protect themselves from body fluids, but their children are not being told anything about pro-

tection and the school is not using any precautions, they see a double standard. These people are not ignorant and stupid, but there is confusion. (*American Medical News*, at 34 col. 1, September 25, 1987)

The two differing approaches appear to be a conflicting message about the risks of acquiring HIV infection, but more accurately represent the difference between risk management, with its emphasis on elimination of as many risks as economically possible, and risk evaluation, or the prediction of probable transmission of infection.

A number of studies have examined the risk of acquiring HIV infection through ordinary household contact, both in ordinary family settings and when increased exposure to blood and body fluids is common, such as in families of hemophiliacs undergoing home transfusions. These studies unequivocally demonstrate that, absent sexual contact, or other, independent, high risk behavior, ordinary daily contact is not associated with any increased risk of acquiring HIV infection. Even among health care workers, who are much more likely to be exposed to infectious material than individuals in the ordinary course of daily activity, the chances of acquiring infection are small unless there is an accidental needlestick or equivalent blood-to-blood contact, and are very low even then. The infectivity of HIV seems to be variable, so that even parenteral exposure is not certain to produce infection. While the occasional report of transmission by activity not ordinarily considered "high risk" means that no one can guarantee the absolute safety of an environment, the overwhelming evidence is that daily social and workplace contact is safe.

Consequently, the assurances of public health officials that HIV infection is difficult to acquire in the absence of sexual or parenteral contact are accurate. HIV infection cannot be acquired by touching, social kissing, coughing, sneezing, or by sharing eating utensils, water fountains, toilet facilities, swimming pools, gymnasiums or other public facilities.

Risk managers, however, must be involved in evaluating educational and workplace environments for the elimination of as many potential risks as economically reasonable, and are consequently sensitive to any situation which is liable to present either an increased chance of injury or an increased potential for lawsuit. They must, as a result, be aware of the ordinary situations in which the risk of infection is increased because of the potential for contact with infected blood or body fluid, and respond in a manner which may be more cautious than that absolutely necessary for the general population. A remote risk for transmission is still a risk, and should be addressed in appropriate policy measures which are proportionate to the problem. Examples of everyday contact which present an increased risk of exposure to infected materials include housekeeping personnel handling bloodied linens or sanitary napkins, special education workers caring for children who cannot control biting behavior, and physical education teachers who must deal with bleeding injuries. Any situation which presents the potential for contact with blood or body fluids presents a theoretically increased risk for HIV infection over casual, everyday contact which does not involve exposure to blood or body fluids, and each environment must be individually evaluated for potential risks. However, experience indicates that, although an increased risk is real whenever exposure to blood or body fluids occurs, it is still not large with the exception of certain well defined and easily identified activity. HIV infection remains an extremely remote possibility absent sexual contact, drug abuse, transfusion of infected blood products or birth to an infected parent.

Chapter V

Public Health Laws

A need for a public body to respond to conditions which pose a threat to the health of society at large was recognized in the latter part of the nineteenth century. State public health departments had been generally established by 1910, when cases addressing the role and propriety of quarantining infected persons began to establish the proper limits of government regulation of personal medical care for public health reasons (Fox, 1986). The role of public health departments has continuously been shaped by a conflict in social and personal values about the propriety and necessity of government intrusion in matters of health. Conflict between personal privacy and autonomy and the right of the public to control threats to its general well being have long been recognized, but the validity of some public health measures as a result of exercise of the state police power is inevitable. That the state may exercise its police powers in the public interest, even the public health interest, so long as its efforts are reasonable, was quickly recognized by the U.S. Supreme Court (*Jacobsen* v. *Moss*).

Currently, each state establishes its own public health laws, which regulate the kinds of diseases thought to represent a public health risk, and the appropriate responses which can be made. The cornerstone of public health management is disease surveillance. All states maintain lists of diseases which must be reported to the appropriate public health authorities. In addition, there are federal regulations mandating reporting of particular diseases through the local public health departments as a condition for receipt of federal funds (42 C.F.R. 51b. 401 *et. seq.*). The reporting of disease serves a twofold purpose: it provides an index of disease activity for epidemiological research and it provides a means by which the state can insure treatment of infected individuals (Gostin, 1986). The methods and motives of the public health system have varied through the years, being subject not only to scientific but social and political pressures as well. Nevertheless, it is a system of reporting, tracking and treatment which was historically implemented and which survives as the basis of public health management today.

VENEREAL AND COMMUNICABLE DISEASES

Statutory approaches to disease reporting and control take two basic approaches. Diseases are classified as either venereal (or sexually-transmitted) or as communicable. Communicable diseases are infectious diseases which may be transmitted from one individual to another. Venereal diseases are communicable, but are more narrowly defined as customarily or exclusively transmitted by sexual means.

Reporting of both venereal and communicable diseases may be mandated by statute. A disease may be classed as a venereal disease by compliance with a statutory definition, because of designation by a state agency responsible for such definitions or by specific listing within the body of the controlling statute. California, for example, defines "venereal disease" as "syphillis, gonnorhea, chancroid, lymphopathia venerea and granuloma inguinale." [Cal. Health and Safety Code §3001 (West 1985)] New York defines sexually transmitted diseases in terms of a list issued by the Commissioner of Public Health. [New York Public Health Law 2(n) (McKinney 1985)]. After the recognition of AIDS as a venereally transmitted disease, some states have incorporated it, and ARC and/or HIV infection into their statutory schemes. [Fla. Stat. §384.23 (1986)]. Some state commmissioners have also included AIDS in their designated list of venereal diseases, but in one case the commissioner refused requests by physicians that AIDS be included. The basis of the refusal was that designation of AIDS as a sexually transmitted disease would give local public health officers too many broad powers, including the traditional powers of quarantine. The commissioner felt that exercise of these powers in an unbridled fashion would impede the accepted policy underlying the approach to caring for AIDS patients (*New York State Society of Surgeons* v. *Axelrod*). Thus, the designation of AIDS as a venereal or communicable disease is not without controversy and may have profound effects on the manner in which the state chooses to follow and attempt to control the disease.

Currently, AIDS is considered a venereal disease only in a few states (Gostin, 1986); in others it is classed as a communicable disease or as a "special problem or unusual" disease, dangerous to the public, according to the standard reporting scheme (Curran II, 1986), or it may not satisfy any particular statutory definition at all (*District 27 Community School Board* v. *Board of Education of City of New York*). Currently, reporting requirements in all states, and federal guidelines, require only reporting of cases of full-blown AIDS as defined by the current CDC criteria and/or AIDS-Related Complex (ARC). Silent HIV infection is not presently required to be reported to the CDC, but a few states require reporting of HIV positive patients regardless of symptoms (Curran I, 1986).

Venereal disease statutes generally provide for contact tracing and treatment of both the index case and discovered cases based on the index report of contacts. Venereal disease statutes provide an automatic basis for state intervention because of identified infection, such as isolation or quarantine. Under communicable disease statutes, isolation and quarantine may be instituted only if state regulations are amended to include the specific disease (Gostin, 1986). All public health statutes provide some protection of confidentiality for diagnosed individuals, although stricter controls are the rule in venereal disease statutes.

ISOLATION AND QUARANTINE

Isolation of infected individuals is the separation of infected individuals from the uninfected population to prevent the transmission of disease. Quarantine is the separation of exposed but not necessarily infected individuals from the unexposed population for a period of time sufficient to determine whether infection has actually occurred, in order to prevent transmission of disease. In order to be effective, quarantine must be for a period equal to the longest possible incubation period of the disease. Both methods have been used successfully in the past to reduce the incidence of freely communicable disease, particularly when no treatment or vaccine was available and control of the spread of disease was largely on a behavioral and population basis. Quarantine and isolation are obviously immense intrusions on personal liberty. Historically, the courts have held that reasonable quarantine measures are permissible as an exercise of state police power even in the face of constitutional safeguards of personal autonomy and privacy (Merritt, 1986). However, these historical quarantine cases were largely decided prior to the definition of modern privacy rights. Modern constitutional interpretation emphasizes privacy to a greater degree, requiring substantial justification for any state intrusion.

It is not entirely clear, however, just what level of judicial scrutiny would be applied to broad quarantine laws. Traditionally, strict scrutiny has been reserved for laws which impair fundamental rights or are based on suspect classifications of race, alienage or national origin. Strict scrutiny requires demonstrating that the law in question be shown to advance a compelling state interest by the least restrictive means, and almost insures invalidation of any quarantine law so examined. AIDS patients do not constitute a suspect class, however, and after the decision in *Bowers* v. *Hardwicke* [106 S.Ct. 284 (1986)], which upheld a sodomy statute, finding it did not impinge on protected privacy interests, it is possible that the right to privacy will not automatically invoke strict scrutiny. Quarantine statutes do, however, impair the right to travel, which is recognized as a fundamental right, and on that basis, strict scrutiny might apply.

An intermediate level of scrutiny, reserved for cases involving restricted access to public education or "quasi-suspect classes" such as sex or identification as an insular minority with a history of discrimination, requires that legislation be substantially related to important government interests. AIDS patients, because of the large proportion of drug abusers and homosexuals, could conceivably be considered such a "quasi-suspect" class. However, in at least one case involving isolation and quarantine, the standard of review was the minimal "rational basis" test, which requires only that the action be rationally related to advancing a legitimate state interest. (*Cordero v. Coughlin*) This case upheld isolation of AIDS patients in prison; however, the court noted that the liberty interests of prisoners are already substantially limited which may limit the applicability of this case to other situations. Despite disagreement about the proper method of review of these statutes, there is considerable doubt among commentators whether any quarantine program can be sufficiently narrowly drawn to be constitutional.

In the case of a disease with a short and defined incubation period, isolation and quarantine will be useful for interrupting the spread of infection only if the disease is relatively freely communicable by casual contact. Historically, however, courts have required that isolation and quarantine applied on a reasonable basis be based on a sound, although not unassailable, medical foundation (*Wong Wai v. Williamson*). Efforts at quarantine which seemed to be based on racial or geographic prejudice were not permitted even before the current climate of deference to individual rights (*Jew Ho v. Williamson*). Even the exercise of a valid state interest in protecting the public health may be unconstitutional if it is not applied with equal vigor to all citizens, and targets only a small population which is susceptible to prejudice.

Thus, current suggestions for isolation and quarantine of patients with AIDS or other HIV infection are untenable on several grounds. The intrusion on personal liberty required by such measures would be much greater than most isolation and quarantine procedures in the past, and there is little scientific evidence that such measures would be effective in controlling the spread of disease.

Because HIV infection is life-long, any proposed isolation would be life-long as well. In the case of a disease not freely communicable by casual means, the balance of the intrusion on personal liberty is too great to allow isolation as a general method for preventing spread of HIV infection. Although there is historical precedent for lifetime isolation of individuals infected with communicable disease (*Kirk* v. *Board of Health*), it is unlikely that such general, enforced isolation would be constitutionally permissible today.

Further, because HIV infection is not freely communicable in the manner that has usually caused the state to enforce isolation and quarantine methods, there is no medical basis for its use as a general measure in containing the AIDS epidemic. Modified isolation or quarantine because of specific behavior, however, may be more defensible, if based on case-by-case analysis and limited to situations in which no alternative method of preventing transmission is available or acceptable. The reluctance of some HIV infected individuals to alter their sexual lifestyle or to inform sexual contacts of the risk of intercourse has been demonstrated. "Patient Zero", for example, a homosexual flight attendant thought to be the first patient to introduce HIV infection to the United States, reportedly continued to have unprotected intercourse for the nearly four years he suffered from AIDS before his death, despite efforts of his physicians and counselors to alter his behavior. Patient Zero is said to have had hundreds of sexual contacts before his death; the implications of such unrestricted behavior in the spread of the infection are obvious (Schilts, 1987).

Some state statutes have anticipated a limited use of these methods by authorizing confinement of individuals unwilling to modify their behavior to prevent infection of others. Limited quarantine based on behavior will also face constitutional challenge, in part because it depends on predicted future, not present, activity. The Public Health Service has only cautiously endorsed the concept of even limited quarantine "only in rare circumstances and after due process" (Coolfront Report). Although there are immense practical difficulties in implementing even modified isolation in the case of HIV infection, it may be a viable public health measure in extreme and very limited cases.

COMPULSORY VACCINATION

All states have compulsory vaccination procedures for entry into public schools. The validity of these laws has been upheld by the Supreme Court, though vaccination cannot be compelled if the life of the individual might be endangered (*Wong Wai* v. *Williamson*). Exemption from vaccination is generally provided for by statute or regulation in cases where vaccination poses a health risk to the individual. In individuals infected with HIV who demonstrate immune compromise, vaccination against common childhood diseases may be ineffective because of inability to form antibodies; or hazardous, if live virus vaccines are used since uncontrolled infection may develop. Guidelines drafted by the Center for Disease Control and the American

Academy of Pediatrics (CDC) should be consulted for a list of situations in which vaccination should be waived. Proper administrative policies regarding compulsory vaccination for students should reflect awareness of the problem of vaccinating HIV infected individuals and provide proper policies for deferral or modification.

CRIMINAL PENALTIES AND HIV INFECTION

Theoretically and practically, criminal law has already entered the arena as one force shaping the public health response to HIV infection. Criminal prosecutions for knowing, attempted transmission of infection by biting, spitting and throwing blood (*People* v. *Richards, People* v. *Prairie Chicken, Indiana* v. *Haines*), attempted contamination of food with HIV infected blood (*Florida* v. *Dunn*), and knowingly selling infected blood (*California* v. *Markowski*) have been instituted.

Knowing intercourse of an individual infected with venereal disease is a misdemeanor under a number of public health laws (Field, 1987). Some states have recently incorporated provisions authorizing testing of convicted prostitutes for venereal diseases [Fla. Stat §796.08 (1986)]. Matters of proof and policing under such laws present obvious problems including the considerable concern that this gives unlimited license to public officials to control and intimidate drug abusers, homosexuals and prostitutes (Field, 1987). Nevertheless, criminal laws may provide an additional method of social control in the most extreme cases of irresponsible personal behavior.

Chapter VI

Discrimination Law and AIDS

One of the most critical questions faced by school and college administrators has become that of when an HIV infected individual can be excluded from the class or the residence halls, or whose attendance or residence may be conditioned on modification of the usual classroom experience. Officials are faced with balancing the needs of the infected student against the fear and concern for the safety of uninfected students which has given rise to so much discrimination against people with AIDS.

That individuals afflicted with AIDS, or simply infected with HIV, suffer from societal discrimination is indisputable. HIV infected individuals have been excluded from housing, the workplace, schools, and public transportation systems. They have suffered abuse and ostracism and have been the objects of violent protests and even death threats. The proposed enrollment of an HIV infected student, when known to the parents of other students, can become a lightning rod for protests and disruption which extend far beyond the institution itself and may persist even after the matter of enrollment is officially resolved. For this reason, HIV infected individuals will seek the protection of federal and state laws prohibiting discrimination.

In the early days of the epidemic, the uncertainly about the applicability of the law of discrimination to people with AIDS, as well as the lack of scientific information to assess the real risk of transmission in the classroom environment, forced many school systems to adopt the policy that HIV infected students would be excluded unless a court, having heard the evidence on the problem, ordered otherwise. In the ensuing years, almost without exception, courts have ordered mainstream enrollment of HIV infected children, generally under the Vocational Rehabilitation Act of 1974 or similar state laws. As the position of the law has become very clear, and as scientific evidence mounts that HIV infection is not transmitted by normal classroom activities, it is no longer wise for schools or colleges to adopt blanket policies excluding HIV infected students. It is a virtual certainty that the court will order admission of an HIV infected student, and the court has occasionally required institutions to go to great lengths to accommodate the infected student. Seeking a court order will now be costly, not only in terms of time and publicity, but also in damages, as students seeking admission who are forced to secure it by court intervention are being awarded damages well into seven figures. Few educational institutions can afford such a financial drain. It therefore behooves the policymakers to understand the basis of discrimination law as it applies to AIDS.

CONSTITUTIONAL PROTECTIONS

The constitutional basis for prevention of discrimination lies in the Fourteenth Amendment, which provides for "equal protection" under the law. Equal protection challenges require state action; they do not apply to truly private situations. State action may be implied in many ways.

State operated educational institutions are clearly within the state action designation for purposes of the Fourteenth Amendment, and thus, local elementary and secondary schools, as well as state colleges and universities, may face fourteenth amendment challenges to their AIDS policies. Private schools present a more difficult problem. For a private institution to satisfy the state action requirement, the state must be significantly involved in the conduct complained of. Mere receipt of funds, licensing or general regulation by the state is not enough (*Moose Lodge No. 104* v. *Irvis*). The courts will generally examine five different areas to determine whether a private school's policy represents state action: receipt of state aid, the extent and intrusiveness of state regulation, whether such regulation connotes approval of the action, whether the school serves a public function as a surrogate for the state, and the legitimacy, on more general grounds, of the claims that the institution is "private" (*Weise* v. *Syracuse University*).

The mere existence of state regulations governing schools is not sufficient to make a private school an arm of the state for purposes of the Fourteenth Amendment (*Powe* v. *Miles*). Nor are state standards regulating the minimum qualifications necessary for a degree (*Grafton* v. *Brooklyn Law School*) or the general review of degrees granted by the state (*Sament* v. *Hahnemann Medical College*). Likewise, although private schools which supply higher education are performing a service which is also administered by the state, this alone does not constitute providing a public function as surrogate for the state which is required by the courts (*Grafton* v. *Brooklyn Law School*).

28

The receipt of financial aid is critical in determining state action but in itself is not determinative. If state funds are a sufficient proportion of the institution's budget, state action is likely to be inferred. In this regard, a university deriving 33% of its budget from state revenues fell under the state action guidelines (*Braden* v. *University of Pittsburgh*) but another receiving 3% of funds from state sources did not (*Weise* v. *Syracuse University*). Tuition supports and scholarships which are given directly to students are not generally sufficient, by themselves, to bring a private institution within the purview of the Fourteenth Amendment.

Other state interactions with private institutions may sufficiently entwine the institution to create state action. Of particular importance are state and municipal leases of land or buildings (*Hammond* v. *University of Tampa*).

Passed after the Civil War, the Fourteenth Amendment was drafted to eliminate racial discrimination against blacks, predominantly in the post-war South. Whether or not discriminatory treatment resulting from state action of identifiable groups is permissible under the Fourteenth Amendment depends largely on whether the group involved composes a "suspect" classification, akin to race, for which the broadest protection is reserved.

The suspect classes include race, national origin and alienage (*Korematsu* v. *United States*, *Graham* v. *Richardson*, *Oyama* v. *California*). If unequal treatment of classes is based on a suspect classification, it can be permitted under equal protection analysis only if it is the least restrictive means to achieve a compelling state interest (*Dunn* v. *Blumstein*). In practice, no state practice which receives this form of strict judicial scrutiny is upheld.

Conversely, if discrimination is based on a classification which is not suspect, such as wealth, unequal treatment is permissible if it is a rationally related method of advancing a legitimate state aim. This is the "rational basis" test, which is the least demanding standard of review. Early public health cases were judged by this standard, which is easily met and rarely invalidates any state action. An intermediate analysis, which requires an important state objective, is applied when the group involved is a "quasi-suspect" classification.

This intermediate level of scrutiny is applied to insular minorities with a history of discrimination, and has also been applied to the right to public education (*Craig* v. *Boren*). An argument for application of this standard to AIDS cases lies in the fact that people with AIDS, homosexual or not, represent a minority against whom discrimination is common.

Even though "rational basis" analysis rarely results in invalidation of state policies, the intermediate level of scrutiny may. Discrimination based on infection by HIV is based on the fact of infection, or, more insidiously, on sexual preference. Neither has been deemed a suspect classification by the court, so that protection from discrimination against HIV infected individuals on constitutional grounds alone may be limited (*Constitutional Rights of AIDS Carriers, 1986*).

If a school is covered by the Fourteenth Amendment, its discriminatory policies may be challenged under the civil rights enforcement statutes (42 U.S.C. 1983). Not only does this guarantee a federal forum for the plaintiff, the statutes provide for substantial damages to the successful plaintiff as well as the payment of attorney fees in addition to the award of damages.

THE VOCATIONAL REHABILITATION ACT OF 1974

Section 504 of the Vocational Rehabilitation Act of 1974 provides that:

> no otherwise qualified handicapped individual . . . shall, solely by reason of his handicap, be excluded from participation in any program receiving federal financial assistance. [29 U.S.C. 794 (1980)]

Thus, under the terms of the act, a handicapped individual may not be denied access to a federally funded program solely on the basis of his handicap, as long as the individual is "otherwise qualified." An individual who is "otherwise qualified" is one who "is able to meet all of a program's requirements in spite of his handicap" (*Southeastern Community College* v. *Davis*), or one who can "perform the essential functions" of a specified job [45 C.F.R. 84.3Z(k) (1985)].

Determination of "otherwise qualified status" is often particular to the situation under consideration; general rules are difficult to formulate. The courts have determined that the inability to fulfill a formal job requirement is not sufficient evidence that an individual is not "otherwise qualified," unless the formal requirements of the job are in reality necessary for satisfactory performance of the job. An essential job requirement is one which is uniformly required of all individuals performing the same function. The courts will sometimes go to extraordinary lengths to insure that requirements which seem reasonable on their face are in fact, essential requirements before determining that an individual is not "otherwise qualified." Thus, for example, in the case of a paralyzed police officer terminated because he could not effect a forceful arrest or render emergency aid, the courts required that a determination be made whether these requirements were in fact necessary for employment as an officer and required uniformly of all active policemen (*Simon* v. *St. Louis County*). Conversely, mental instability with suicidal tendencies is sufficient to render a mental health counselor unqualified (*Doe* v. *Region 13 Mental Health-Mental Retardation Committee*) and vertigo may be the basis of excluding an individual from the position of aerial photographer (*Caylor v. Alabama*).

If an individual is not otherwise qualified because of his handicap, accommodation of the handicapped individual by the program is an affirmative obligation, so long as it does not present undue hardship on the program, if such accommodation will allow the handicapped individual to meet the qualifications of the program. Accommodation ceases to be reasonable when financial and administrative burdens become excessive (*Southeastern Community College v. Davis*), or when it fundamentally alters the nature of the program [45 C.F.R. 84.22 (1985)]. The requirement of accommodation may include making available alternative placement which is usually available under customary practices.

DEFINING HANDICAP:
School Board of Nassau County v. Arline

The definition of handicap under Section 504 is:

Any person who (i) has a physical or mental impairment which substantially limits one or more of such person's major life activities, (ii) has a record of such impairment or (iii) is regarded as having such an impairment. [29 U.S.C. 706 (7)(b) (1980)]

Physical impairment is:

any physiological disorder or condition, cosmetic disfigurement, or anatomical loss affecting one or more of the following body systems: neurological, musculoskeltal, special sense organs, respiratory, including speech organs, cardiovascular, reproductive, digestive, genitourinary, hemic and lymphatic, skin and endocrine. [45 C.F.R. 84.3(j)(2)(i) (1986)]

Major life activities include caring for one's self, performing manual tasks, walking, seeing, hearing, speaking, breathing, learning, and working [45 C.F.R. 84.3 (j)(2)(ii)].

Whether an infectious disease qualifies as a handicap under the Vocational Rehabilitation Act was questionable prior to the decision of the Supreme Court in *Arline* (*School Board of Nassau County v. Arline*). Gene Arline was a teacher with a past history of tuberculosis. When she suffered a recurrence of her disease, requiring hospitalization, she was relieved of her teaching duties and ultimately fired. Arline argued that her discharge was wrongful under the act because it was based solely on the fact of her illness, which qualified her as a handicapped person entitled to reasonable accommodation by the school board. The Supreme Court ultimately agreed, establishing that an infectious disease qualifies as a handicap under the Rehabilitation Act.

The Court pointed out that Arline's illness certainly impaired her life activities, since it affected her lungs and required hospitalization.

Because there were insufficient findings of fact by the trial court, the case was remanded to determine whether, in light of the handicap, Arline was otherwise qualified to perform her duties as a teacher. In this way, the decision in *Arline* is limited, holding merely that an infectious disease may be considered a handicap, thus triggering the requirements of the Rehabilitation Act of determining the issues of "otherwise qualified" and whether reasonable accommodation can be made, if not.

The contention of the school board was that Arline was fired, not because of her handicap and its effect on Arline herself, but because of fear of transmission of the infection to others. The Court indicated that the contagious effects of a disease must be considered part of the handicap itself, particularly since the purpose of the act is to prevent irrational discrimination because of the fear or revulsion a handicap produces in other individuals. Discharge from a teaching condition might be justified, if supported by legitimate concerns about significant health and safety risks. Such risks must be supported by sound medical opinion, based on:

(1) the nature of the risk (how the disease is transmitted);
(2) the duration of the risk (how long is the carrier infected);
(3) the severity of the risk (what is the potential harm to third parties);
(4) the probability that the disease will be transmitted and will cause varying degrees of harm.

Infectivity and handicap must be determined on the basis of sound medical testimony in each individual case. Further, the Court indicated that great deference would be given the opinion of public health officers. It declined to indicate what, if any, weight would be given to private medical opinion relied on by the employer in making his decision. It is probable that the opinions of public health officers and the pronouncements of the CDC will be accorded the greatest weight and will, in essence, determine the issue of medical judgment. Any private physician will be faced with the necessity of proving expertise in the area of HIV infections but may have the advantage of being the only individual familiar with the particular facts of the individual situation. However, given the recent criticism of the handling of the AIDS crisis by public health officers (Schilts, 1987), the opinion of government officers, while important, may no longer be unassailable.

Following the logic of *Arline*, it did not take long for AIDS and ARC to be formally recognized by the court as handicaps under federal law, and subject to protection under The Rehabilitation Act (*Chalk v. United States District Court, Doe v. Centinela Hospital*). In addition, many state laws and regulations also recognize AIDS as a handicap (*Shuttleworth* v. *Broward County; Cronan* v. *New England*

Telephone). *Arline* does not offer blanket protection prohibiting discharge or exclusion of individuals with AIDS, although in light of present knowledge, the risk of transmission by usual work or classroom activity is so small that individuals will be protected. Rather, it emphasizes that determinations of "otherwise qualified" and "reasonable accommodation" must be individual, and may vary with the facts of any particular case. *Arline* defines, albeit vaguely, the factual inquiry which must enter into a sound medical determination which can support exclusion on the basis of risks of transmission. In the questionable or borderline case, the determination must be on an individual basis.

The finding of *Arline* has been codified in the Civil Rights Restoration Act of 1987 (Pub. Law 100-259), which provides:

. . . for purposes of (sections) 503 and 504 (of the Vocational Rehabilitation Act of 1974), as such sections apply to employment, such term does not include an individual who has a currently contagious disease or infection and who, by reason of such disease or infection would constitute a direct threat to the health or safety of other individuals, or who, by reason of the currently contagious disease or infection, is unable to perform the duties of the job.

The impact of this language is to clarify that individuals who have infectious diseases are protected by the Rehabilitation Act, so long as they pose no threat by their presence under the *Arline* criteria. It also seems to indicate that employers are not obligated to hire infected individuals when they are not otherwise qualified by reason of their infection, or when other legitimate considerations, not within the scope of the act, would support a refusal to hire or retain the individual. Although no cases have been determined on the basis of this new statute, it appears from the face of the provision that it is confined to employment situations.

Arline specifically declined to answer whether HIV infection in an asymptomatic individual qualifies as a handicap. Because silent HIV infection produces no effect on major life functions, it may technically not fulfill the statutory definition of handicap. An argument can be made that even the silent infection of an individual is a handicap because of the adverse social effect and general response of the public to anyone infected with HIV. In this regard, HIV infection is like cosmetic disfigurement: the effect on the individual may arise more from the misperceptions of individuals around him than from the disease itself. Extending the protection of the Rehabilitation Act to asymptomatic carriers of HIV is in keeping with the intent of Congress and the court to prevent irrational discrimination based on fear and replace it with responses grounded in reasoned and sound medical judgment. Subsequent rulings have borne out this intent as the asymptomatic carrier state has been recognized as a handicapping condition in the absence of having full-blown disease with adverse physical effects (Doe v. *Centinela Hospital*).

Handicapped individuals probably cannot be excluded from a program because of fear of future complications, such as the fear of increased job absenteeism because of infections (*Chrysler Outboard Corp.* v. *Dilhr*). State court decisions, under state laws similar to the Rehabilitation Act, have held that evaluation must be based on present ability to perform a task, rather than on fear of future incapacity. However, if the risk of future incapacity is significant enough, it may render an individual unqualified (*E.E. Black Co.* v. *Marshall*). It has been suggested that an employer might justify a refusal to hire on the argument that he should not be required to hire and train an employee destined to die in a relatively short period (Cecere, 1987). In the case of the individual with full-blown AIDS, the likelihood of survival is indeed short, generally a year or so following diagnosis, and incapacity may be great, although an increasing number of patients with full-blown AIDS are surviving for longer periods and with less debility because of advances in treatment. However, in the case of silent HIV infection, there is no way to reasonably predict life span in any individual and thus, this argument fails.

In the context of education, the potential application of this argument is probably limited to long term, high cost educational programs, such as medical school or other advanced degree programs, and to employees in the system who require long training and would need to have a long tenure to make the investment in training cost-effective. Most classroom situations and training programs clearly do not fall into this category, and the possibility of relatively rapid turnover of students and staff is routinely accepted.

Likewise, fear of higher insurance costs is irrelevant (*Chrysler Outboard Corp.* v. *Dilhr*). In addition to the general protections provided by the Rehabilitation Act, many state laws address the provision of insurance to HIV infected individuals and prohibit, to one degree or another, either the use of HIV testing at all in underwriting or limit its application to certain situations, such as high policy limit life insurance policies. This varies from state to state, and local laws must always be consulted.

State laws governing discrimination against the handicapped also afford protection for victims of AIDS. A significant number of states have rendered administrative decisions which classify AIDS as a handicap for purposes of state law, including California, Colorado, Florida, Maine, Massachusetts, Minnesota, Missouri, New Hampshire, New Jersey, New Mexico, Oregon, Washington and Wisconsin (Parmet, 1987). Additional protection against discrimination is also afforded by specific state laws prohibiting the use of HIV testing in determining employment, housing or insurance (U. S. Department of Health and Human Services: Current Status of Law on AIDS). Many of the state statutes prohibiting discrimination against HIV infected individuals track the language of Section 504, thereby making the provisions found in the federal law equally applicable to all individuals within the state without regard to federal funding.

OTHERWISE QUALIFIED AFTER ARLINE:
Application of the Rehabilitation Act To People With AIDS

Arline clearly established that the Rehabilitation Act applies to individuals handicapped because of infectious disease, and indicated that the effects of the infection could not be isolated from the handicap. It detailed the fact that determination of qualification on the basis of infection must rest on sound scientific grounds, whether examining physical infirmity or the risk an infected individual poses within the environment. Taken together with the cases decided before *Arline* which detail the process by which an individual may be determined to be "not otherwise qualified," some relatively clear guidelines emerge.

The determination of "otherwise qualified" for purposes of the Rehabilitation Act will permit assessment, even after *Arline*, of the risk to others the infected individual presents in the school or work environment. It seems clear that when the infected individual presents a significant risk to others, he is no longer "otherwise qualified." Thus, blood donors who are HIV infected are legitimately excluded from the donor pool. *Arline* leaves open how great the risk of transmission need be to render an individual no longer qualified. Previously, the courts had indicated that a significant medical risk, though not necessarily one exceeding 50%, must be present to render an individual not otherwise qualified (*Doe* v. *New York University*). Thus, it appears that there theoretically may be situations in which an HIV infected individual, despite the relative lack of transmission of disease, may not be otherwise qualified for particular positions, whether in school or employment.

Only in rare cases, however, has the court been willing to find AIDS or HIV infection alone a significant enough risk to render an individual not otherwise qualified. The extremely low probability of transmission during ordinary activity in the usual classroom setting means that virtually no classroom environment will present a significant risk of transmission. Recent cases involving the admission of HIV positive students confirms this general attitude. In reaching their decisions, courts have relied heavily on the statements of policy and health care issued by the CDC.

CDC guidelines indicate certain situations in which some restriction of enrollment may be appropriate because of increased risk of transmission. Incontinent children and those who cannot control biting behavior, or who have sores which cannot be adequately covered, represent a slightly increased risk of transmission because of increased exposure to body fluids. Accordingly, an HIV infected student presenting these features might be rendered "not otherwise qualified," although at least one court has determined, in contradiction to the rather firm CDC statements, that essentially no risk of transmission is presented by such children in the classroom and has ordered admission (*Thomas* v. *Atascadero*).

Students or employees in positions which themselves present an increased risk of parenteral exposures between individuals, such as catheterization labs or dialysis units, are a group which might represent a significant risk under the *Doe* rule, although the risk of transmission is still well below 50%. The CDC has considered that these individuals might be appropriately screened for the presence of HIV infection, and has debated whether it is appropriate to exclude such individuals from the workplace if such invasive procedures are required. No firm position has been adopted, however, and it seems unlikely that, in the absence of such a firm declaration the courts will find a significant risk for purposes of determining an individual "not otherwise qualified."

In summary, it appears that the presence of HIV infection alone will virtually never render an individual not otherwise qualified for enrollment or employment under the guides of the Rehabilitation Act. Blanket rules of exclusion, therefore, are not viable.

HIV infection, even without the presence of full-blown AIDS, however, may present sufficient health problems that the individual is not otherwise qualified based on the effects of the disease, though not on the infection alone. Such a determination must take into account not only the bona fide requirements of the task, but the usual procedures for handling those who do not or cannot meet them. In the employment situation, the focus should be on the actual job requirements, physical and emotional.

For example, an employee who is chronically absent from work is not otherwise qualified, whether the absenteeism is based on HIV infection, alcoholism or a recent divorce. Properly documented, such absenteeism is a permissible basis for discharge, as long as the policy is evenly administered to all who violate it.

Likewise, students suffering HIV infection who are sufficiently fatigued may not be able to participate in sports programs. If brain infection has resulted in erratic and uncontrollable behavior, a student may not be qualified for classroom participation in the same way that severely emotionally disturbed children are not. Thus, in determining the issue of "not otherwise qualified" in the HIV infected student, focus must be on the *effects* of the infection rather than on the fact of infection itself. Ample precedent supports the exclusion of individuals, who cannot meet bona fide qualifications, from job and classroom situations.

The analysis of qualification for students follows the same logic as does that of determining employment qualification. The actual requirements for enrollment must be examined in the same way as bona fide job qualifications, and the policies for dealing with those who do not meet the requirements must be evenly applied. In many situations, the only "qualification" of a student is the ability to be present and attentive in the classroom. Further qualifications may apply to particular activities, such as labs or physical education. The administrator must be wary of using physical infirmity as an excuse for exclusion actually based on the fact of HIV infection. Because accommodation of handicapped children is routine in all school systems, defined in part by the Education for All Handicapped Children Act (see below), routine policies for meeting the needs of the handicapped must be extended even-handedly to HIV infected students as well.

Paternalistic policies which are enacted for the student's own health or safety, and against his wishes, are also risky. In the case of AIDS, this concern has special applicability, because HIV infection is associated with a high susceptibility to common infection which may become life threatening in the HIV infected person. School environments offer great exposure to these highly communicable diseases, such as chicken pox and meningitis. Reasonable accommodation, as well as common sense, dictates that schools provide alternative educational programs for those children who cannot participate in the classroom setting when there is a likelihood of infection. Thus, it is appropriate to provide home schooling for HIV infected students during periods of epidemic illness, and a system should be in place to notify parents of prevalent infections which cause an increased risk to the HIV infected student. It is not viable, however, to use the fear of infection as a basis for excluding HIV infected students from the classroom at all times or against their informed wishes at any time. If the student chooses to remain in a situation which presents personal risk, but for which he is otherwise qualified, after being presented with alternatives, school policy cannot force exclusion (*Poole* v. *South Plainfield Board of Education, Wright* v. *Columbia University*).

In general, for both student and employee, the determination of qualification must be made in the present, not the future. HIV infection predisposes to infirmity and early death, but because of the extreme variability in incubation period and ultimate expression of the disease, little can be predicted with certainty in regard to the course of infection in any particular individual, even when symptomatic disease is present. Thus, in the absence of already existing manifestations which render an individual not otherwise qualified, the probability that a handicap will develop because of HIV infection is probably not sufficient to render an individual not otherwise qualified.

In contrast to this general rule, the court has indicated one particular situation in which future infirmity and medical needs might be sufficient to render an individual not otherwise qualified under the Rehabilitation Act. The case involved a foreign service officer whose medical condition required access to care not available at all stations to which he might be posted overseas. Because government policy required foreign service officers to be available to be posted anywhere in the world, a finding of not otherwise qualified was merited and upheld (*Local 812 of Government Workers* v. *United States Department of State*). Thus, for schools and colleges which offer foreign study programs, especially in places where parasitic and communicable diseases are particularly prevalent and health care is limited, exclusion of HIV infected students may be supported on the basis of this particular exception. It is important to note, however, that this case involved government agents and qualification for important government service, not elective participation in a school program. An attempt to restrict HIV infected students in a similar manner from private participation in foreign study may be analyzed, not under this logic, but as a paternalistic policy generally is. Any such policy must be carefully scrutinized to avoid discriminatory intent and practice. Alternatives, such as providing detailed information to students who elect to participate in programs which place them at risk and obtaining appropriate releases rather than unilateral exclusion of particular groups, should be strongly considered.

In summary, caution, common sense and the law dictate that policies which ultimately act to exclude any individual from school participation be drawn on the basis of discernible, present effects which themselves render the individual unqualified, not on the basis of the underlying afflictions which produce the effects. Because the proper focus of the Rehabilitation Act is on the ability of the individual to perform required functions, objective examination of skills and qualifications, without regard to the individual disease process which restricts abilities, allows the drafting of policies which are equitable and less likely to run afoul of the Rehabilitation Act in all areas, not just the matter of HIV infected students. A great variety of afflictions may produce the same disability which renders an individual not otherwise qualified. A policy which focuses on the effect and not the disease is less likely to result in disparate treatment of different individuals with the same actual disability.

WHEN DOES THE REHABILITATION ACT APPLY?
Federal Aid After Grove City

The provisions of the Rehabilitation Act do not apply to truly private institutions which receive no federal aid. The extent to which the Rehabilitation Act applies to educational institutions receiving federal money is the subject of some debate.

Under the decision of the court in *Grove City College* v. *Bell,* only the programs of a school which receive federal funds are subject to the provision of the Rehabilitation Act. Under this rationale, policies which are discriminatory under the Rehabilitation Act are permissible as long as they are not applied in programs which receive federal money.

This led to the somewhat contradictory result that academic institutions which received federal money could discriminate in parts of the academic program, so long as they were willing to forgo federal money in funding that particular program. Congress has now effectively repealed the decision of *Grove City* by passing the Civil Rights Restoration Act of 1987 (Pub. Law 100-259) which extends the protection of the Rehabilitation Act to cover all programs in an institution which accepted federal funding in any part. Although a portion of the act codified the *Arline* decision with respect to infectious diseases (see above), this appears to be limited to the employment situation. The statute is sufficiently new that no cases have arisen to test the extent of the change, but it appears that, except for some limited employment situations, receipt of federal aid of any sort in any school program will render the entire school subject to the provisions of the Rehabilitation Act.

EDUCATION FOR ALL HANDICAPPED CHILDREN ACT

In an attempt to provide practical funding to insure equal access to public education for handicapped children, Congress passed the Education for All Handicapped Children Act (EAHCA) in 1975 [20 U.S.C. 1401-1461 (1975)]. Under EAHCA, handicapped children are defined as "mentally retarded, hard of hearing, deaf, speech or language impaired, visually handicapped, orthopedically impaired, or other health impaired children, or children with specific learning disabilities who by reason thereof require special education and related services." Under the act, these children are entitled to specially designed instruction at no increased cost to the parents, including instruction at home or in a hospital if necessary, and including transportation and other related services. EAHCA, by its provisions and intent, fosters mainstreaming of children as an important goal. EAHCA provides that to the extent appropriate, children, including children in public or private care facilities, are educated with children who are not handicapped and that special classes, separate schooling or other removal of handicapped children from the regular educational environment occurs only when the nature or severity of the handicap is such that education in regular classes with the use of supplementary aids and services cannot be achieved satisfactorily.

The degree to which a handicapped student must be accommodated under EAHCA can be considerable. Among the provisions the court has required to be made have been schooling during summer sessions, transportation, in-class aides to assist handicapped students, and special physical facilities to accommodate physical disability.

EAHCA operates by requiring specific state action in order to obtain federal funding. States must insure that, to the maximum extent possible, handicapped children are educated in a regular classroom environment, with non-handicapped children, unless to do so precludes satisfactory education (*Campbell* v. *Talledega County Board of Education, Johnson by Johnson* v. *Ann Arbor Public Schools*). Contagious diseases will qualify as handicaps under EAHCA if they compromise a child's ability to perform in the classroom setting because EAHCA covers "other health impaired children," as long as the disease poses no significant risk of transmission to other children. Without the demonstration of health impairment, it would seem that silent HIV infection of the asymptomatic carrier is beyond the scope of EAHCA.

Mainstreaming children with infectious diseases such as hepatitis B, similar in transmission patterns to that of HIV infection yet far more freely transmissible, has been upheld by the court (*State Association for Retarded Persons* v. *Carey*). It is thus likely that, under EAHCA as under the Rehabilitation Act, any grounds for excluding or limiting the student must be based on sound scientific principles and not on unwarranted concern for transmission in an unlikely setting.

Under the EAHCA analysis, children with AIDS may be considered handicapped (Bodine, 1986). EAHCA is particularly important to schoolchildren because of its requirement of mainstreaming the handicapped child whenever possible, effectively excluding isolation as a routine policy for these children unless supported by medical evidence. Significantly, if EAHCA applies, it is the exclusive remedy available, and requires that a child seeking admission exhaust administrative remedies before seeking judicial resolution of his claim (*Smith* v. *Robinson*). This requirement reflects the preference of the courts that such disputes be resolved, whenever possible, at the local level, but it may mean lengthy local procedures and hearings. For example, in one of the earliest and most famous cases seeking admission of a student with AIDS, Ryan White sought admission to school. His case was decided on the basis of EAHCA because he was already symptomatic with AIDS. Ryan White was initially denied access to school in Kokomo, Indiana, in 1985. Although he ultimately won admission in February 1986, he was again barred from attending for seven months while the court determined whether he fell under the provisions of the state communicable disease act. It was ultimately determined that AIDS was not a communicable disease within the definition of the act, and Ryan was allowed back in the classroom, but not before he had been excluded from the classroom for the great majority of the school year.

SUMMARY:
Admissions and Restrictions of HIV Infected Students
HIV infected students are clearly protected under the Rehabilitation Act, EAHCA, and similar state laws regarding discrimination against handicapped individuals. Thus, in almost no circumstance will blanket exclusion of HIV infected students, symptomatic or not, be permissible. The presumption of the institution's policy must be that HIV infected students are qualified to be enrolled. Attention may then be focused on individual students and situations to determine the legitimate qualifications for participation which must be met. If any student, HIV infected or not, fails to meet these legitimate qualifications and cannot be reasonably accommodated, exclusion from the program is permitted.

The extent to which accommodation must be made can be very great. A recent case ordering mainstream enrollment of an HIV infected child with severe retardation and behavioral problems required the isolation of an HIV infected student within a specially constructed plexiglass booth in a regular classroom as reasonable accommodation to her handicap. This, of course, requires construction of a permanent facility, the specifications of which were outlined in great detail by the court (*Martinez* v. *Hillborough County School Board*). Administrators will be faced with substantial demands on the part of parents who want their children enrolled and must be prepared to meet some extraordinary requirements to satisfy the demands of reasonable accommodation.

The threat of transmission, in most situations, will not be sufficient to restrict a student's attendance in the regualr classroom. A small theoretical risk of transmission will not be sufficient to outweigh the detrimental effects to the student of exclusion from the classroom (*Chalk* v. *District Court of Northern California*). If a verifiable, scientifically sound increase in the risk of transmission arises, either because of the infected student's medical condition, or the activity in which he is expected to participate, restriction may be reasonable if based on sound medical evidence. Administrators should be cautious in this area, however, since very few school situations will qualfiy as present-

41

ing an increased risk of transmission which is appreciable. Those which do, may often be managed by sound environmental policies applied equally to all participants, leaving, again, very few situations in which exclusion or restriction of the HIV infected person, on the basis of fear of transmission, will be supportable.

Policies which assist HIV infected individuals in assessing their personal risk in participating in school activity should be adopted, and administrators should be careful that all students and their parents are properly aware of what risks exist in various activities. Paternalistic policies which exclude students from full participation in activities because of concern for the student's health will be suspect and should be avoided when possible.

The same principles which define the proper weight given HIV infection in determining school enrollment also apply to employees. Rarely will HIV infection alone be sufficient to render an individual not qualified if the Rehabilitation Act or similar anti-discrimination laws apply. As a result, the proper focus of inquiry should be on the physical and mental abilities of students and employees, without regard to the underlying medical condition which produces them. When a bona fide inability to meet the essential functions of a job or classroom environment exists, and accommodation is not possible or reasonable, the afflicted individual may be legitimately excluded. If no inquiry is made about underlying diseases, such as HIV infection, which produces the pertinent disability, no claim can be sustained that discrimination is actually being based on impermissible concerns of transmission or because of inherent bias against HIV infected individuals.

Chapter VII

Confidentiality and Limited Disclosure

Because of the social implications of a diagnosis of HIV infection, concern for confidentiality has emerged as a central issue in the AIDS crisis. Because of the ostracism and persecution associated with identification, often erroneous, as a homosexual or drug abuser, the public's unwarranted fear of contagion and the mistaken impression of much of the general public that AIDS is a "gay disease," civil liberties groups and gay rights associations have lobbied strongly for increased guarantees of confidentiality in protection of HIV test results. Public health officials have expressed concern that inadequate guarantees of confidentiality, or programs of mandatory testing, will drive high-risk individuals "underground," effectively eliminating the opportunity to diagnose, treat, educate and counsel HIV infected individuals fearful of negative social responses. Yet management of AIDS as a disease, and control of the current epidemic also requires acknowledgment that the uninfected population may sometimes have a legitimate right to know about the presence of HIV infection. Public health law dealing with the control of infectious disease has always required a balance between personal privacy and preeminent societal concerns about the management and exposure of infection. The AIDS crisis has brought to the attention of the public and the courts alike the inherent, and largely unresolved, conflict between insuring personal rights to confidential treatment of medical information and the legitimate interest of the public to be free of unnecessary health and safety risks.

Thus, in a broad social sense, public concerns about information pertaining to the prevalence and incidence of HIV infection must be balanced against personal rights of privacy and confidentiality. The weight of legal opinion and the thrust of most newly drafted statutes has been to emphasize the confidentiality of the infected individual, largely because of the extremely low risk of transmitting the disease in casual settings. For educational officials, this means that information about HIV infection is most likely to be considered confidential, and unauthorized disclosure will subject the school or college and its officials to civil liability for breach of confidentiality and invasion of privacy. The situations in which a third party will have a sufficient interest to warrant disclosure of information over the objection of the infected student will be very rare.

CONFIDENTIALITY OF MEDICAL INFORMATION

Either by statute or common law, all states protect the confidentiality of medical information, whether the result of a private doctor-patient relationship or one arising between school physician and student. Modern medical ethics maintains physician-patient confidentiality as integral to the physician-patient relationship. The American Medical Association Code of Medical Ethics states that:

A physician may not reveal confidences entrusted to him...unless he is required to do so by law or unless it becomes necessary to protect the welfare of the individual or community. (AMA Principles of Medical Ethics Article 9)

Note, however, that this does not mandate strict confidentiality in all circumstances, but contemplates the existence of circumstances which justify disclosure contrary to a patient's wishes.

State statutes, regulations and case law also protect the confidentiality of written medical records, as do the requirements of the Joint Commission on Acreditation of Hospitals. The Privacy Act of 1974 [5 U.S.C. 552(a) (1977)] applies to protect the confidentiality of records in federal institutions or rendered by federal contractors. This includes government hospitals, government contracting health maintenance organizations, and even institutions with federally funded registries.

The general standard for confidentiality of patient medical information is that it may not be disclosed to any third party without consent of the patient; to do so in the absence of justification gives rise to a cause of action for damages which result from the disclosure. In the case of unjustified disclosure of HIV infection, damages have sometimes been significant: loss of employment; personal suffering from social estrangement; loss of insurance benefits; even, occasionally, loss of home and belongings.

Such a breach of confidentiality gives rise to liability under a number of theories: breach of fiduciary duty; breach of statutory duty of confidentiality; and invasion of privacy (Lamb, 1983). Justification for release of otherwise confidential information, in the absence of patient consent, is a defense to an action for breach of confidentiality. Justified release of information has historically been defined under several specific situations in which courts have deemed that third parties have sufficient interest in medical information to outweigh lack of consent from the patient himself to excuse disclosure of the information.

JUSTIFIED DISCLOSURE TO THIRD PARTIES
Disclosures Required by Statute

Despite the strict dictates of medical confidentiality, there exist in all states some statutory exceptions to protection of medical information. Disclosure to public health authorities, for example, is justified on the basis of a statutory duty imposed on the physician who is required to report certain diseases. All states require the reporting of AIDS, though most do not require notification by patient name. A few states mandate, in addition to the reporting of AIDS cases, reporting of all HIV positive individuals. Colorado requires reporting by patient name (United States Department of Health and Human Services, *Current Status of Law Regarding AIDS*). In addition, some states have enacted laws requiring reporting of infectious diseases in some circumstances of known exposure to infection, such as notifying emergency transport personnel who have given emergency care to HIV infected patients [Fla. Stat. section 395.0147 (1987)].

Statutory justification of disclosure of HIV infection is limited. Public health authorities to whom information is disclosed are required to maintain confidentiality of the information under specific state laws mandating confidentiality, often in detailed and specific terms. Public health laws provide substantial safeguards for confidentiality and public health officers are generally conscientious in their protection of patient identity (Fox, 1986). Florida, for example, prohibits disclosure of public health information except by court or statute, or to protect a *named* individual in a medical emergency [Fla. Stat. section 384.29 (1986)]. Other states have similar provisions.

Disclosures Of Risks To Public Health

Even early cases recognized that personal rights to confidentiality must occasionally give way in the face of overriding public concern. Thus, there extends a line of cases from the early part of the Twentieth Century which establish that unauthorized disclosure of medical information may be made when the patient poses a risk to the public health.

The seminal case in this regard is *Simonsen* v. *Swenson,* which involved a patient who was diagnosed with secondary syphilis. The patient had large numbers of open sores by which the infection could be freely transmitted to others by physical contact. The patient's physician advised that the patient give up his lodgings in a public hotel, and when he did not, advised the landlord of the patient's condition.

Despite the fact that the patient ultimately was proved *not* to be suffering from syphilis or any other contagious disease, the disclosure by the physician was upheld as proper under the circumstances. The court found that disclosure was based on a reasonable (although erroneous) diagnosis, and the risk of contagion, had the diagnosis been accurate, was both real and significant enough to outweigh the patient's interest in confidentiality of his medical records.

These cases establish that unauthorized disclosure of medical information is appropriate when the physician believes that disclosure is reasonably necessary to prevent the spread of disease; the disclosure is limited to those who would otherwise be exposed; the diagnosis and disclosure are made on reasonable grounds and in good faith; and the disclosure is not malicious. The language of the court in defining the circumstances in which disclosure is permissible makes it clear that only limited disclosure to legitimately exposed individuals at significant risk of contracting disease is contemplated:

> no patient can expect that if his malady is found to be of a dangerously contagious nature, he can still require it to be kept secret from those to whom, if there were no disclosure, such disease would be transmitted. If the patient's disease is found to be of a dangerous and highly contagious nature that it will necessarily be transmitted to others unless the danger of contagion is disclosed to them, the physician should, in that event, if no other means of protection is possible, be privileged to make so much a disclosure to such persons as is necessary to prevent the spread of the disease. (*Simonsen* v. *Swensen*)

Not only is the risk of contagion (risk of transmissibility) emphasized, but also the seriousness of the disease itself, recognizing that the more serious the disease, the less acceptable is any significant risk of transmission. Most current discussion of confidentiality concerns in HIV infections focus only on the risk of transmissibility, assuming it to be low, and ignoring the critical emphasis of these cases on the potential severity of disease if in fact it is transmitted.

In the case of HIV infection, significant risk of transmission is largely limited to sexual partners, and those who might come in contact with blood or body fluid of the infected person. This would include needle sharing addicts, health care workers and potential recipients of blood or organ and tissue transplants. Because HIV infection has been identified with transplantation from an infected donor, as well as treatment with growth hormone derived from autopsy harvested pituitary glands, the interest of organ procurement agencies in determining the HIV status of donors is substantial. Many donors are recent accident victims who have received sufficient blood transfusions to "dilute out" a positive HIV antibody in their own blood, making it even more critical that procurement agencies have access to alternative information about a donor's HIV status, if it is available.

Disclosure might be justified to family members or roommates who are at risk for exposure to blood and body fluids or needles beyond that normally found in cohabitation. This might include individuals undergoing home dialysis or treatment with clotting factors for hemophilia, especially if the household contains individuals too young or otherwise incapable of understanding and avoiding the risk associated with blood contact or needlesticks. Most adults, however, will not fall into this category, and the abundance of studies indicating that household exposure results in no increased risk of transmission makes disclosure to household contacts risky in the absence of patient consent.

Sexual contacts are almost certainly within the scope of the *Simonsen* rule, because the risk of transmission from unprotected sexual activity is extremely high. State laws, however, may limit the applicability of *Simonsen*, by limiting the protection for unauthorized disclosure to disclosure to the spouse of an individual. This results, in part, from the suggestion that sexually active individuals within high risk groups must be aware of the risk of transmission even without specific warning, and should conduct themselves accordingly.

In general, the position that individuals must learn to conduct their daily lives to avoid exposure to HIV infection without specific information is both accurate and admirable. However, the theoretical risk of HIV infection because of high risk behavior is still much less than the very real and present possibility of transmission by intercourse with an individual known to be infected. Further, even in the infected individual, there is evidence that limiting exposure to the virus may mitigate the effects of infection. It is currently unsettled when unauthorized disclosure may be made to sexual contacts other than a spouse. In specific medical situations, the decision is often made on moral grounds, and carries the very real possibility of liability for breach of confidence. For colleges facing the reality of sexual activity in residence halls, the prudent course is a policy which does not contemplate the disclosure of such information; coupled with a policy of explaining to students the facts about HIV infection and transmission and a firm, unequivocal statement that information about students who are infected with HIV will not be disclosed to friends, classmates, roommates or known or potential sexual contacts.

Although there exist workplace situations in which the risk of transmission may be increased, generally, the workplace is a sufficiently casual environment that transmission is not a substantial risk, and therefore, disclosure to co-workers would not ordinarily be justified. Exceptions, for example in health care fields, must be based on CDC policy and should be narrowly drawn. In any case in which disclosure of information to an interested third party is contemplated, permission should first be sought for the disclosure, and the HIV infected individual should be encouraged to participate in the disclosure himself. In some states, this is a requirement for protection under statutes limiting liability for unauthorized disclosure to a spouse or in other circumstances. Local statutes should always be consulted and legal advice sought when particular situations fall outside the defined scope of state statutes.

Disclosures To Interested Parties

One spouse has traditionally had a legitimate interest in the health of the other, and disclosure of medical information has been permitted on this basis, based at least in part on the legal anachronism that a husband and wife are one during marriage (*Curry* v. *Corn*). Disclosure has been allowed in the midst of divorce proceedings (*Mikel* v. *Abrams*) and has even been extended to a fiance when marriage has not yet taken place (*Berry* v. *Moench*). However, if information is sufficiently sensitive, such as that gleaned from psychiatric care, it may not be legitimately subject to disclosure, even to the spouse, in the absence of physical danger (*MacDonald* v. *Clinger*).

The employment relationship does not automatically give rise to a legitimate interest in the health of an employee. The employer who wishes to obtain medical information about an employee must be prepared to demonstrate that his interest is justifiable because the medical condition has a bearing or effect on the discharge of duties, rather than on some employer-imposed requirements for employment (*Horne* v. *Patton*). In the case of HIV infection, more often than not, the employer has no legitimate interest in the employee's infection *per se* (*See* Chapter 6, *supra*). Some situations, however, will provide a sufficient nexus to allow employer interest to be recognized. An employer involved in a workers' compensation claim, for example, has a legitimate interest in medical information relating to that claim and the employee, by filing a claim, has put his physical condition at issue (*Acosta* v. *Carey*).

Balancing of the employee's right to privacy against the employer interest, has been suggested as a standard for evaluating disclosure in cases of legitimate employer interest in medical information, conforming with the general approach to determining the appropriate limits of patient confidentiality (*Bratt* v. *IBM Corp.*). Nowhere is such a balance more critical than those circumstances in which co-worker or other third party safety may be compromised because of the effects of disease on an employee, even in the absence of a likely transmission of the disease.

The recognition of AIDS dementia brings this problem to the forefront. Central nervous system effects are being increasingly recognized in the course of HIV infection, and range from depression to confusion and forgetfulness, to outright psychosis, and in extreme cases, coma preceding death. HIV induced dementia may develop in advance of other symptoms of AIDS.

The recognition that HIV infection may compromise mental acuity has implications for the potential disclosure of medical information. In patients who demonstrate neurological impairment because of the virus, counseling and behavior alteration may be unsuccessful because of inability to comprehend the significance of the disease, or because of the development of dissociative mental changes. In severe cases, involuntary guardianship or other civil commitment procedures may be necessary because of severe incompetency.

In some work environments, the risk of any condition which alters concentration, mental acuity or judgment cannot easily be tolerated because of the potential of harm to co-workers and other third parties: public transport workers, workers in nuclear plants, air traffic controllers, government workers with high level security clearances. In such situations, employers may have a legitimate interest in any condition which results in decreased performance. These jobs are particularly sensitive because the first "on the job" mistake may cause considerable injury or loss of life. Thus, the physician who identifies HIV associated (or any other) dementia in patients with such sensitive jobs must decide whether the level of impairment is sufficient to present a safety risk to others. It is not clear when disclosure under such circumstances is mandatory, but it may be discretionary if sufficient safety concerns are present.

However, the dictates of discrimination law limit the circumstances in which employers may legitimately inquire about the presence of HIV induced neurologic changes in the absence of some documented, job-related failure to perform adequately. Further, potential future incapacity is probably not a sufficient ground for discharge or limitation if the Rehabilitation Act or other anti-discrimination laws apply. Blanket policies are not likely to be legitimate, but those tailored to positions in which public health and safety are likely to be compromised may be acceptable. Cases such as *New York City Transit Authority* v. *Beazer* imply that public health and safety concerns must take precedence over privacy and employment rights when a real risk of potential injury exists, but the limits of this, especially within the confines of the evolving AIDS epidemic, have yet to be defined. In *Beazer*, the New York City Transit Authority was permitted to exclude narcotics addicts and individuals on methadone programs from certain safety-sensitive positions, despite the dictates of the Rehabilitation Act of 1974. In the case of HIV infection, safety sensitive posi-

49

tions may be limited to those in which the CDC ultimately concedes that seropositivity is a disqualification, if indeed any exist. At the present, none have been so designated, although suggestions have been made that health care workers who do intensive invasive procedures such as cardiac catheterization may represent a population in which screening and limitation on the basis of seropositivity may be appropriate. Otherwise, the effects of HIV infection on job safety relate more to the effects of disease on the individual than to infection itself. Consequently, strict physical qualifications for such safety sensitive positions as bus driver, as well as routine and regular examinations to detect developing handicaps which compromise job performance, regardless of source, are more useful as policies than attempted blanket exclusion of individuals on the basis of HIV infection.

JUSTIFIED DISCLOSURE: Duty To Warn

Most justifications for unauthorized disclosure provide a defense for elective disclosure of medical information made in the discretion of the physician because of mitigating circumstances. However, in some circumstances, if the risk to third parties because of non-disclosure is sufficiently great, unauthorized disclosure becomes a duty owed to the third parties at risk. The seminal case describing this "duty to warn" is *Tarasoff* v. *Board of Regents of the University of California. Tarasoff* established that, despite a physician's duty to maintain confidentiality of patient information, there is an affirmative duty to warn third parties of a risk of injury once it has been determined to exist. The case involved a psychiatric outpatient who indicated to his physicians that he intended to kill a university student, his former girlfriend. The psychotherapists contacted the police, who picked up and interviewed the patient and determined independently that he was not dangerous. The patient was released, and subsequently murdered the student. The California Supreme Court ultimately upheld the contention of the family that the psychotherapists, having once determined the patient to be dangerous, owed a duty directly to the potential victim to warn her of the death threat.

The duty to warn is in direct conflict with the individual right to privacy, and courts have not always been clear in deciding how the balance between personal privacy and public safety must be struck (Stone, 1976). The duty to warn is predicated on a "special relationship," in *Tarasoff*, between physician and patient, sufficient to trigger a duty to third parties. Other such special relationships are that of: parent and child (or school, when in *loco parentis*); landowner and licensee; individuals in charge of those with dangerous propensities (usually health and psychiatric workers); and in some cases, law enforcement officers; schools and teachers in relationship to those under their control (Rest. 2d. Torts sections 315-320). In most instances, the cases following and expanding on *Tarasoff* have limited the duty to warn to situations of physical danger from psychiatric patients who have threatened third parties. The majority of courts require that a known risk be identified to a specific third party, and decline to establish a duty to warn a "large, amorphous" group of potential targets (*Thompson* v. *County of Alameda, Lipari* v. *Sears, Roebuck, Brady* v. *Hopper*). Most cases involve intentional torts, such as battery, rather than exposure to risk of injury or disease. Even when applied outside these limits, courts have held that it is necessary for the physician to make a reasonable determination of potential dangerousness, as well as have available some definitive protective measure, in order to raise a duty to protect an individual or group at risk.

It is clear that the *Tarasoff* duty has some application in the case of individuals with HIV infection, although there is disagreement about the action it requires. Some commentators suggest that the duty to warn be limited to medical professionals; and that it can be satisfied by advising the patient to notify sexual contacts and observe proper standards of behavior (Gostin, 1987). Only if grounds exist to suspect non-compliance would the physician be required to take further action. Such an approach is extremely sensitive to the privacy concerns of individuals infected with HIV, but misapprehends the impact of the *Tarasoff* decision. The duty to warn is an independent duty which is owed to a third party independent of, and in conflict with, the duty of confidentiality owed to a patient. Once a physician duty to warn arises because of the existence of a threat to the health of a third party, it must be satisfied by steps, adequate and reasonable under the circumstances, to warn or protect, if possible, the individual at risk. In light of this, it is questionable whether counseling of the HIV infected contact will suffice to satisfy the direct duty to warn a known third party at risk. However, counseling may be independently required, either by the dictates of state statutes, or the duty of the physician to make sure the infected individual is aware of the side effects of his disease and its treatment (*Kaiser* v. *Suburban Transportation System*). Failure to inform a patient of side effects which ultimately result in injury of a third party, such as neglecting to tell a bus driver that medication he takes may cause drowsiness which ultimately results in an accident and injury to a third party, may be actionable as negligence. This, of course, requires that injury to third parties is sufficiently foreseeable (*Duvall* v. *Golden, Kaiser* v. *Suburban Transportation System*). In the case of HIV infection, transmission in the usual classroom situation is remote. The potential for passage of infection in residence halls or because of recognized illicit drug use is probably foreseeable, but may be beyond the control of school officials except for general educational efforts aimed at informing the student population about the medical facts concerning AIDS and HIV infection. The individual physician or counselor, whether or not operating in a school setting, has a clear duty to attempt to educate his HIV infected patients about the possibilities of transmitting infection to others, and the steps which must be taken to minimize or eliminate the risk.

The extent to which the duty to warn will be extended to educational administrators and teachers is as yet unsettled. Although teachers and school officials are in a "special relationship" with students, their duty to protect students stems largely from the inability of students to otherwise defend themselves from risks, or from forced association with individuals likely to harm them, found in the educational environment (Rest. 2d Torts 320). Associational risks are generally those from which the individual cannot be expected to protect himself, and require anticipation of risks likely to develop before they in fact occur. These principles, along with the fact that HIV infection is generally unlikely to be transmitted in the usual educational environment, limit the circumstances under which a school or college may legitimately disclose HIV infection of a student. In addition, courts have been reluctant to impose a duty to warn on the basis of infectious disease, refusing to find a duty on the part of health professionals to warn of epidemic outbreak of communicable disease with a relatively low infectivity, though still much more communicable than HIV infection, such as hepatitis B, or the presence in the community of a carrier of such a disease (*Gammil* v. *United States; Derrick* v. *Ontario Community Hospital*). Because general principles of public health and hygiene are designed to limit the transmission of disease, even in the absence of knowledge of particular risks, and because personal habits of hygiene and care are most effective in preventing the spread of disease when uniformly complied with, this result is a sensible one. Ultimately, the responsibility of the individual must be to develop sound personal health habits which are self-protective. This posture has been adopted by such agencies as the American College Health Association (Keeling, 1986), and is reflected in a growing number of school board policies addressing the issue of disclosure.

Adopting the position that, ultimately, it is a personal responsibility to develop health habits which protect against spread of HIV infection concurrently raises a duty to provide students with sufficient educational opportunities and information about AIDS, and its transmission, to be able to protect themselves adequately. The development of age-specific programs which teach the essentials of preventing HIV transmission: avoidance of blood and body fluids, proper disinfection of wounds and spills of such infectious materials, safer sexual habits and avoiding drug use must be implemented at all levels of education and repeated consistently to have an impact on the AIDS epidemic.

PUBLIC RECORDS LAWS

State colleges and universities, and public schools are subject to public records laws which vary from state to state, but which to one degree or another, allow public access to information generated or received in the course of conducting business. Consequently, materials which contain sensitive material about students may be accessible because of public records statutes, leaving educational officials liable for breach of confidentiality.

The confidentiality of student records, mental health records and health records is frequently guaranteed by state statutes, exempting such records from the provisions of public records laws. Thus, individual records require consent before they may be released to or examined by third parties. Any information contained in student files which are educational records, mental health or medical records is deemed confidential and protected under public records laws.

However, memoranda, reports, committee minutes and general correspondence, if made in the course of business are potentially public documents subject to inspection and copying on demand. The inclusion of otherwise confidential information in such documents leaves a school potentially in breach of confidentiality and liable for invasion of privacy. Thus administrators in state and public schools should be especially wary of including information about HIV status in materials which might be construed as public records. Disclosure of HIV infection of a student by office memorandum, for example, may involve a public document which might provide the basis for civil liability.

Specific communication about HIV infection should be kept to a minimum, and, whenever possible, specific names or other identifying characteristics avoided. Particularly if no legitimate purpose can be served by having the information, as is often the case, administrators should seek to avoid receiving or retaining sensitive information.

School committees which are designed to assist HIV infected students are compromised by the requirements of public records laws. In order for such committees to function properly, confidentiality of the students and their families must be insured. However, if improperly conducted and designed, the communications of such a committee may be considered public records and subject to public inspection. Maintaining the records as medical records is one avenue to help insure confidentiality. As "educational records" under the Buckley Amendment, proceedings may also be confidential. Certainly, any committee dealing regularly with HIV infected student status and handling sensitive information should be internally designated as confidential. The growing number of states which have chosen to enact statutes guaranteeing the confidentiality of HIV test results lends support to this position. If public access to potentially confidential information is sought, a refusal to supply until competent legal advice, even to the extent of a declaratory judgment, is obtained is the best way to avoid the liability which results from unauthorized disclosure.

STUDENT RECORDS: The Buckley Amendment

In schools and colleges which receive federal funding, the confidentiality of student educational records is insured by the provisions of the Family Educational Rights and Privacy Act of 1974, also known as the Buckley Amendment. This statute provides that written permission from the parent or the eligible student is necessary before information in the record can be released. It further provides that the student and his parents must have access to the student's records, which was previously often denied by school officials before passage of the Buckley Amendment, and mandates a procedure under which challenges or corrections to the student record can be made by the student or parent. For the purposes of the Buckley Amendment, federal funds are broadly defined as direct and indirect assistance, including student loans and work-study programs.

Under the Buckley Amendment, educational records include information compiled by the institution which is relevant to student activity, even if the information is not contained solely within the individual student file. Disciplinary records, even those of campus security, testing reports, counseling reports and health information are all within the scope of educational records under the Buckley Amendment. Private notations of administrators or educators about particular students are not considered student records if they are retained by the individual who makes them and not revealed to others, except for substitutes (Baker, 1987). Confidentiality provided by the Buckley Amendment exempts some school records from the provisions of public records laws, but the conflict between the provisions of state and federal laws on the subject has not been entirely resolved by the courts. Because state laws vary considerably on the issue of public records, student records are best considered potentially protected under the Buckely Amendment, except to those individuals who can demonstrate a proper interest in them (*Young* v. *Armstrong School District*). When determining whether to include sensitive information in student files, it is wise to consider the record open to public scrutiny, not seeking or retaining unnecessary information which, if disclosed, would result in liability. On the other hand, when determining whether to release information without authorization, it is more prudent to assume the record will be protected. Needless to say, specific facts will alter the legal decision in any given case.

The Buckley Amendment provides for disclosure of student information without authorization only in limited situations. Student information may legitimately be disclosed to school officials and teachers with a legitimate interest in the subject matter (*Palladium Publishing Co.* v. *River Valley School District*). Thus, school officials may legitimately exchange relevant information about HIV infection in the process of planning for and accommodating special needs of infected students, and may communicate with proper medical and public health officials. Caution should prevail, however, because often the fact of infection is irrelevant to properly providing for the handicapped HIV infected student.

Under the Buckley Amendment, and in keeping with the legal philosophy of *Tarasoff*, unconsented disclosure of educational records is appropriate in emergency situations when a significant risk of harm exists. Because of the low communicability of HIV in nearly all classroom settings, unauthorized disclosure of HIV status is almost certainly not within the scope of the emergency exception to the Buckley Amendment. The Buckley Amendment acts as potential protection against suits claiming injury for failure to warn. Any suit brought against a school alleging that a student became infected with HIV because of failure to warn of the presence of another HIV infected student in the classroom, may be successfully defended on the basis that the requirements of the Buckley Amendment prohibit disclosure. This approach has been successfully asserted in cases involving students whose dangerous behavioral tendencies fell within the protection of the Buckley Amendment, and in which, causation was much more clearly established than is the case with room transmission of HIV (Baker, 1987).

Chapter VIII

Tort Liability For
Diagnosis and Transmission
Of HIV Infection

Tort liability for HIV infection follows general tort law principles including those of negligence and privacy law. However, the volatile nature of the AIDS epidemic and the peculiar nature of the infection have put established law in a new light. In many cases, competing legal duties create a legal "Catch-22:" it is not always possible to chart an entirely safe course of conduct to avoid all potential liability when confronted with the reality of juggling the interests of an HIV infected individual, the demands of the school or workplace and the legitimate concerns of third parties. In some measure, risk management of tort liability with respect to the AIDS epidemic has become a question of which suits one prefers to risk and potentially defend.

It has become clear that two major areas of liability for educational institutions have emerged: liability for illegal discrimination on the basis of handicap; and for breach of confidentiality or invasion of privacy for improper disclosure of information about the status of students infected with HIV. In the few years that AIDS has become a significant issue in the public eye, the dictates of law in these areas have become rather well defined, and the risks of non-compliance are well recognized and substantial. Accordingly, schools and colleges should devote a good portion of their energies to insuring that their policies and actions fall within the defined limits imposed by anti-discrimination and confidentiality statutes.

Less significant in terms of legal risk but more troublesome in terms of individual conscience is the matter of insuring that schools do not present an environment in which HIV infection is facilitated or actively transmitted. Fortunately, the biology of HIV infection makes this a remote possibility. Still, many administrators harbor fears that the educational institution may ultimately be charged with liability should a student or employee claim that HIV infection was acquired as a result of school contact, particularly if the claim is made that the transmission could have been avoided by disclosure of confidential information.

The role of schools and colleges in educating students about the risks and realities of HIV transmission is only beginning to emerge, but it is inevitable that a duty will ultimately be defined which requires schools, in one measure or another, to provide accurate information to students in order that they be able to protect themselves against the risks of HIV infection. This must ultimately include a duty on the part of schools to keep HIV infected students appraised of situations which, because of the immune compromise presented by HIV infection, are threatening to the HIV infected student himself.

Finally, schools must address the issue of testing and screening. Little has been settled concerning the situations in which screening and testing are appropriate on a large scale, but particularly in colleges and universities which offer health care training programs, educational programs exist in which HIV testing of students may ultimately play a role. Designing such programs to avoid running afoul of anti-discrimination statutes, and maintaining confidentiality of results presents only one aspect of the problem. Testing and screening must be done in a competent fashion with appropriate counseling available if liability for negligent testing is to be avoided.

College affiliated hospitals, blood banks and transfusion services, infirmaries, physicians and other health care providers who must deal with HIV infected patients, known and unknown, face the usual risks of legal liability attendant to patient care. Medical malpractice actions may arise from a failure to diagnose or treat HIV infection; for transfusing contaminated blood products or as a result of a worker's infection from handling infected fluids; for failing to obtain informed consent prior to performing a test for HIV infection or for failing to provide adequate counseling or follow-up once testing is done.

BREACH OF CONFIDENTIALITY

The confidential status of HIV test results has been discussed in detail in Chapter Seven. It is clear that personal medical information is protected by both common-law dictates of physician-patient confidentiality as well as by statutes which provide for confidentiality of HIV test results and of student records. The number of states which provide specific statutory protection of HIV test results is growing, and all require consent, sometimes written, specific and individual, before HIV test results can be disclosed to third parties other than those, such as public health officials, blood banks and organ procurement agencies, specified by law. Even when disclosure is appropriate in light of confidentiality statutes, care must be taken to limit disclosure to those with a legitimate interest.

High profile, indiscriminate communication of a student's infection with HIV, is an invitation to suit. In medical situations, this often occurs by labeling of patient charts with prominent, eye-catching stickers which announce the fact of HIV infection. Similar policies may be employed in school records offices and should be discouraged. Before any school personnel seek access to, or are given, information about a student's HIV status, close consideration must be given to whether there is in fact a need, rather than a mere desire, to have the information. In light of the dictates of anti-discrimination statutes, and the fact that most classroom risks can be handled best by applying simple hygiene precautions universally, relatively few situations will arise in which there is a defensible need to know about HIV infection.

It is advisable, then, for school officials at all levels to consider adopting the position that they will not actively seek information about HIV infection from students, because possession of information related to HIV infection raises a duty of confidentiality. It is foolish to risk the liability of a suit for breach of confidentiality because of information which, ultimately, can serve no legitimate purpose because of anti-discrimination laws. Likewise, if information about HIV infection is received, school officials must limit the retention and distribution of information which is volunteered to the smallest number of professionals possible. Education of school personnel at all levels regarding the dictates of privacy law and the special sensitivity of HIV related information should be a top priority. Hallway consultations, informal discussions and any communication of information about HIV status which cannot be guaranteed the highest degree of confidentiality should be eliminated. Particular attention must be paid to the public records laws, and it should be determined, with as much certainty as possible, which records in the institution are subject to public inspection.

It is clear that there will be situations in which public interest dictates limited disclosure of medical information, even in the absence of consent. Unfortunately, the conflict of public interest and personal privacy is not always clear, and the circumstances in which unauthorized disclosure is clearly permissible are relatively few. Recent trends in the law make it clear that personal privacy is the favored interest in dealing with HIV infected individuals, except when a clear and specific danger of transmission can be demonstrated by competent medical evidence. If a school situation arises in which this seems to be the case, enlistment of local public health officials is imperative. They are likely to be the source of medical expertise which the courts regard as qualified to render judgment on questions of transmission and prevention. Further, within the confines of state public health laws, particularly with respect to medical emergencies, public health officers may have latitude to disclose or to act from confidential information which is denied to school officials themselves.

FAILURE TO WARN

Under the doctrine raised by *Tarasoff*, educational institutions, as well as hospitals, physicians and other health care workers may be liable to third parties who are likely to be exposed to infection because of contact with an individual known to be infected with HIV. Although the current law is unsettled, there undoubtedly are situations in which transmission of disease from a patient to a third party at risk is sufficiently probable that a duty to warn arises. Balancing the confidentiality rights of the infected patient with the duty to warn endangered third parties will prove a difficult task, and one in which the courts have as yet provided little guidance.

Because most school situations provide little real chance for transmission of HIV, in most instances school officials will have no duty to warn. School physicians, because their responsibility to the patient extends beyond the confines of the classroom experience, may find themselves confronted with situations in which a duty to warn becomes a possibility. The liability of a school physician to third parties for failure to warn is predicated on a likelihood of infection in the absence of a warning and a legally sufficient causal relationship between the lack of a warning and contracting the disease. The particulars of this balance are discussed in Chapter Seven. No firm answer exists for the situations in which warning is required, but some states have begun to enact statutes protecting the disclosure to the spouse of an individual in certain circumstances. If it is uncertain whether warning a third party is both appropriate and legally sound, a prudent course is to refer the situation to the local public health officials who may be able to handle the matter as a public health emergency and may be protected by statute for their actions in such situations. Disclosure of information about HIV infection to public health officials is protected by statute, which means that no additional liability is incurred by a school or physician choosing to enlist such assistance in handling a sensitive situation.

EXPOSURE TO INFECTIOUS MATERIALS

Establishment of sound infection control policies which are consonant with current public health recommendations is important in minimizing liability for workers who become infected as a result of exposure to infectious materials. Current AMA and CDC recommendations require that all blood and body fluids be treated as potentially infectious. Simplistically put, "if it's wet, it's dirty." Schools must act to develop sound policies for handling exposure to infectious material and see that such policies for environmental control are both understood and followed. This means providing proper equipment for disinfecting spills in classrooms, adequate supplies of disposable gloves and medical equipment, and policies requiring that open sores of all kinds be adequately covered.

Colleges with curricula including health professions education must insure that students are adequately informed of proper precautions required of health care professionals dealing with patients, including the scope of universal precautions recommended by the CDC. Health care workers must also be instructed in appropriate handling of infectious materials, and adherence to established policy is critical.

Because of the known difficulty in transmission of HIV, even with deep needlestick injuries, a plaintiff exposed to HIV contaminated materials as a result of school exposure may not be able to prove causation if HIV infection is ultimately documented, especially if there has been no pre-exposure HIV test documenting the absence of antibody. This proof of causation is further compounded by the unknown prevalence of silent HIV infection in the population and the extremely long latent periods which the infection may demonstrate, making it possible to acquire the infection prior to or outside of school contact.

Although no one can insure that suits alleging infection because of school exposure will not be filed, most should be successfully defended if proper environmental control policies are in place and followed, because the likelihood of infection under such circumstances is so remote, and exclusion of HIV infected students is not legally permissible.

Health education programs present an increased risk of exposure simply because of their nature. Students entering health professions should be fully appraised of the risks of transmission of HIV in the health care setting, and of the fact that they will be expected to care for HIV infected patients, known and unknown. Written acknowledgment of the guiding philosophies of patient care, the risks inherent in health professions and the prevailing infection control practices is strongly recommended, and should be obtained at least annually.

NEGLIGENT FAILURE TO DIAGNOSE HIV INFECTION

Negligent failure to diagnose HIV infection is actionable under the same circumstances that other negligent failures to diagnose and treat disease are actionable (Hermann, 1987). Schools may be involved if school nurses or physicians fail to recognize HIV infection, and thus fail to refer the student for treatment. University based physicians and hospitals are liable for failure to diagnose HIV infection on the same basis as private practitioners, and may be at greater risk because of the concentration of expertise in treatment of HIV infection in academic institutions. Failure to diagnose may result in aggravation of the patient's underlying condition, directly or as a result of inappropriate treatment being misapplied because of the error in diagnosis.

Because of the adverse social results of a diagnosis of HIV infection, erroneous diagnosis of a patient as infected may also result in liability although there is no direct effect on the physical health. If, for example, employment is denied as a result of testing, there may be a basis for recovery, both on grounds of negligence and because of violation of the provisions of the Rehabilitation Act. Further, because of the personal anxiety which attends a diagnosis of HIV infection, a physician or hospital may be liable to a wrongly diagnosed patient for negligent infliction of emotional distress.

TRANSFUSION OF CONTAMINATED BLOOD PRODUCTS

Liability for transfusion of contaminated blood products is limited to medical schools and the rare situation in which a school physician in a college, university or residential facility might order transfusion of blood for a student-patient. Nearly all states have "blood shield" laws which declare the transfusion of blood to be a service, rather than the provision of a product subject to strict warranty liability (Lipton, 1986). Thus, in the absence of negligence, hospitals, physicians and blood banks are protected from civil liability, as will be schools whose liability is derived from their actions. Care must be taken to insure that blood products are only given when needed, however. If HIV infection results from transfusion which was not medically indicated, and thus negligently given, liability may still result.

Failure to follow accepted transfusion and blood processing guidelines will provide a basis for negligence, but adherence to an inadequate standard is not necessarily a guarantee of immunity if the court decides to impose a stricter standard (*Helling* v. *Carey*). Negligence may result from failure to follow outlined procedures for obtaining, testing and processing blood, from using blood for transfusion before proper testing, for negligent testing, or for transfusing blood in the absence of medical indications. Since the institution of screening procedures, the incidence of transfusion- associated HIV infection has fallen sharply. Occasional cases still occur because of the lag period between infection and development of antibody responses detectable by screening tests. For this reason, negligence may also be alleged on the basis of inadequate efforts to exclude, by alternate means, such as questioning of high-risk donors more likely to transmit infection or failure to institute new test procedures on a timely basis. Although liability for transfusion-related HIV infection is substantially limited by blood shield statutes and requirements of causation and negligence, blood banks are finding it increasingly difficult to obtain liability insurance to cover their activities. Professional staff responsible for transfusion services must keep abreast of current practices and medical review of transfusions, to insure that unnecessary blood products are not administered, will serve to limit institutional liability for these activities.

LIABILITY FOR HIV TEST RESULTS

Aside from the implications of confidentiality statutes, schools must address the desirability of offering or requiring HIV testing of students in limited situations. Colleges and universities can expect that there will be a demand for elective testing for students concerned about their health or potential exposure to HIV. Students in the health professions may request the availability of screening before entering training to establish their baseline status, which is also of interest to the school in terms of defining their potential liability because of HIV infection acquired as a result of contact during the term of enrollment.

It must be remembered that all medical procedures require informed consent of the patient before they may be performed; to perform a procedure in the absence of consent is to risk an action in battery. Most blood tests are routinely performed without elaboration of the risks and benefits attendant to performing the test because the tests are simple, the risks are few and the consent is implied from the fact that the patient has sought the care of a physician in diagnosis and treatment of some disorder. In the case of HIV testing, however, the adverse effects of diagnosis, personal, social, physical and psychological, probably dictate that informed consent, as well as appropriate follow-up and counseling, be a part of the testing procedure. Some states have already passed specific informed consent laws which detail the information which must be given to a patient prior to testing by any individual, whether personal physician or in a school or employment setting. Prudence dictates that HIV tests not be drawn without written consent, including information about the meaning of test results, the availability of counseling and the measures necessary to prevent infection by and transmission of HIV. No test result should be reported as positive without proper confirmation of the test result by a competent laboratory.

Failing to inform a student-patient of the significance of a positive HIV test may result in liability to the patient, or to a sexual partner thereafter exposed. Failure to offer HIV testing to high risk groups, or those to whom a positive test would be significant, may also be negligent. If routine physical examinations are part of a school's programs, especially if performed by school physicians, any information about HIV infection must be passed to the student (or parents) to avoid liability for any resulting transmission which might have been avoided by proper disclosure (*Wojcik* v. *Aluminum Co. of America*).

The impact of the diagnosis of HIV infection is immense. Counseling programs are essential to insure that patients understand the importance of the diagnosis, what precautionary and hygienic measures are necessary to prevent transmission, and to help patients cope with the adverse psychological impact of diagnosis. Cases of suicide and depression following diagnosis have been reported. Thus, any school affiliated medical program which undertakes testing for HIV must also be prepared to deal with this possibility, particularly among college and university students. Long term support through established local support groups, may be instrumental in assisting HIV infected individuals in coming to terms with their disease, and returning to productive life. Local public health offices generally maintain a listing of agencies and groups involved in AIDS support.

Chapter IX

Policies For Environmental Safety

It is incumbent upon all providers of facilities to take all reasonable measures to insure that the environment is safe for those who use it. In the case of HIV infection, this means limiting the potential for exposure to blood and body fluids. In most school situations, this simply means developing policies for management of common, every day accidents providing exposure to blood and body fluids, which can be accomplished by simple methods of disinfection. Very few school situations provide opportunity for parenteral exposure to HIV infected materials, but these situations should be sought out and carefully controlled. If appropriate environmental policies are implemented, the school environment can be made as safe as any other, providing essentially no increased risk for HIV transmission.

GENERAL GUIDELINES FOR
HANDLING BLOOD AND BODY FLUIDS

The recommendations for general precautions to prevent HIV infection because of exposure to blood and body fluids have been developed for use in health care settings. It must be remembered, however, that there is nothing special about the health care environment except the magnitude of exposure which is likely. Blood and body fluids are no more inherently infectious in an emergency room than in a classroom, playground, gymnasium or residence hall; the only difference is the amount and frequency of exposure. Any spill of blood or body fluid should be treated as potentially infectious and handled accordingly. According to recommendations of the CDC, this includes using gloves when cleaning up such spills, and disinfecting with an appropriate agent capable of inactivating the virus. A dilute solution of household bleach (1:10) is sufficient to inactivate the virus. If spills are large, the area should be flooded, cleared and a repeat application of disinfectant applied. If bleach is an inappropriate solution to use because of the potential for harm to the surface (such as carpeting), tuberculocidal disinfectants may be substituted.

Floors and walls are not associated with transmission of infection, since bloodstream contact is ineffective and because the virus is fragile outside the body. Thus, the CDC recommends that no extraordinary attempts are necessary to disinfect these areas, and that disinfectant-detergents registered by the EPA are sufficient if used in a routine manner. Germicides which are tuberculocidal may be used to disinfect spills in areas which may be damaged by application of bleach. There is essentially no risk of transmitting HIV through contact with large surfaces such as walls, floors, and tables. Clean-up of spills, however, involves contact with potentially infectious material, and should be handled accordingly. A proper disinfectant should be employed, and appropriate barrier methods should be utilized. Custodial staff should be provided gloves and proper disinfectants to handle clean up of potentially infectious material. This includes not only spills of blood and other body fluids, but sanitary napkins and contaminated medical waste as well. Education of custodial and support staff about the potential for HIV exposure in handling waste is often overlooked but is of critical importance.

Soiled laundry appears to present a negligible risk of transmission of infection. Contaminated linens should be bagged in leakproof containers. If hot water-detergent washing is used, the cycle should be twenty-five minutes at 71C (160F). If low temperature (less than 70C, 158F) is used, chemicals suitable for low temperature washing should be used according to recommended instructions.

Infectious waste must be recognized by maintenance workers, custodians, students, teachers and administrators alike. This includes any waste potentially contaminated with blood or body fluids and includes such diverse items as sanitary napkins, bandages, and ice packs used to treat bloody sports injuries. These should be bagged in leakproof containers and disposed of properly. In hospitals and other settings in which hazardous and infectious wastes are common, the standard precautions for hazardous and infectious waste should be followed. In other settings, secure bagging of the waste is probably sufficient. The use of gloves by anyone handling wastes should be encouraged to decrease the potential for accidental exposure. Reusable gloves should be regularly cleaned and properly disinfected. Many schools now provide disposable gloves in classrooms for use by students and teachers in dealing with the small accidents that children often have in class, such as nosebleeds, vomiting and "potty" accidents. It is a good practice to provide sturdy, reusable gloves which will tolerate cleaning with bleach for those dealing with infectious material on a regular basis, such as custodians.

Hospitals, infirmaries and other health care environments present particular problems because of the amount of exposure to blood and body fluid which occurs routinely. CDC guidelines prohibit mouth pipetting, and emphasize barrier methods to prevent exposure (gloves, masks and protective eyewear), control of leakage from specimen containers, disposal of waste in accordance with EPA rules and routine disinfecting of laboratory work areas. The same policies and precautions should be implemented in teaching laboratories where blood or body fluids are handled. Laboratory exercises should be drafted to eliminate as much exposure to blood and body fluids as possible. Demonstrations should be confined to competent staff who are well schooled in proper procedures and who can thus avoid unneeded exposures of students. There is probably no place for science experiments involving the use of human blood or body fluids in elementary or secondary schools unless the materials have been pre-screened for the presence of HIV antibody. If blood drawing is required, the phlebotomist should adhere to the routine practices of hospital based phlebotomists, including the use of disposable needles and gloves during the procedure. Needles should never be recapped because of the possibility that accidental needlestick will occur.

Routine sterilization procedures for patient care equipment are sufficient to inactivate the HIV virus. Any instrument which enters tissue, blood or blood vessels must be sterilized before re-use. Instruments in contact with mucous membranes should be sterilized if possible, or receive high level disinfection. This includes dental devices. Those which cannot be sterilized must be disposable or protected by impermeable coverings which may be replaced between uses. These policies should be implemented in teaching clinics as well as regular patient care areas including school clinics and infirmaries.

RECOGNIZING RISKS

Formulating general policies for handling contaminated blood and body fluid is only half the battle. Proper implementation requires recognizing when exposure might possibly occur. Regular review of activities is essential in order to identify and address situations in which blood and body fluid exposure is possible.

Certain situations are predictable, obvious and recurring: cuts and scrapes on the playground or classroom which will be cleaned and dressed by the teacher or in the infirmary, for example. Sports activities are very likely to produce bleeding injuries. Teachers and coaches must be aware of proper procedures to avoid blood contact, including the use of gloves, proper bandaging of bleeding wounds, disinfection of contaminated areas, and the use of disposable items when disinfection or sterilization between uses is not possible. Ice packs should be designed to be used only once, for example. Athletes should be removed from participation when bleeding injuries occur, and until control of the bleeding is obtained, bloody equipment changed or sterilized and the wound bandaged. It should be recognized that, even though blood is potentially infectious for HIV, sweat is not, and no special requirements need be implemented to deal with sweat-soaked clothing, towels or equipment as long as there is no blood.

Rigorous controls should be considered for laboratory and machine shop work, because of the risk of penetrating injury. Proper implementation of general safety rules will reduce the incidence of injury, and hence the exposure to blood. Strict guidelines for performance of any biologic experiment using human blood must be adopted in accordance with CDC guidelines for hospital laboratory work. The risk of transmission from saliva is low, but any activities which present exposure to saliva should be conducted according to CDC guidelines for dental workers: gloves should be worn, and instruments should be either disposable or sterilized.

Ultimately, exchange of blood and body fluid generally occurs in needle sharing (usually drug addiction), blood transfusion, or sexual intercourse. However, other activities may also result in blood contact and transmission of infection: any penetrating injury with a contaminated instrument including tattooing, ear piercing, and accidental needlestick, artificial insemination, and prolonged exposure of broken skin to infected blood. Proper evaluation of the environment for situations analogous to these and implementation of appropriate infection control practices will eliminate the risk of transmission of HIV infection. Blanket policies for infection control form the basis of good environmental risk management, but must be individually implemented with proper attention to the particular activities conducted in the individual environment.

GENERAL WORKPLACE & CLASSROOM GUIDELINES

Because of the low risk of transmission of HIV in the usual environment, most workplace and classroom activities are safe. HIV infection is not transmitted by sharing office space, sitting next to an infected individual, sharing telephones, swimming pools, showers, toilet facilities, eating facilities or water fountains, nor by sneezing, coughing, or nose-blowing. In short, if there is not exchange of blood or body fluid, the activity poses no risk of transmission of infection, and should not be restricted because of fear of transmission of HIV infection.

Chapter X

Accommodating the
HIV Infected Individual

Common sense and discrimination law both dictate that because of the low infectivity of the virus under ordinary circumstances, the HIV infected individual should be allowed to participate in ordinary affairs to the extent possible. It is clear that blanket prohibitions on the activity of HIV infected persons, which do not require individualized assessment of increased risk of transmission, are not generally acceptable. The American Council on Education notes, for example, that:

> . . . schools will be on firmer legal ground if they make decisions on a case-by-case basis with the support of professional medical judgment. (Steinbach, 1987)

CLASSROOM ENROLLMENT OF THE HIV INFECTED STUDENT

Current CDC guidelines recommend that HIV infected children generally be allowed to attend regular classes, as long as they are in control of their behavior and bodily functions. The National Education Association has adopted these recommendations in its recommended guidelines as well (National Education Association). Although challenges to the enrollment of HIV infected children in regular classrooms are relatively frequent, the invariable result has been for the court to order enrollment in the usual classroom setting if the child presents no risk of transmission. Thus, the benefits of enrolling a child known to be infected with HIV only at the order of a court, in an attempt to avoid what is at best a remote liability for the potential transmission of HIV in the classroom setting, are almost certainly outweighed by the adverse publicity which invariably results from such a public confrontation and the near certainty of liability for a civil rights suit following successful forced enrollment. It no longer appears questionable that HIV infected students generally are eligible for enrollment in the regular classroom, and that isolation of HIV infected students is not permissible.

Maintenance of HIV infected students in the ordinary classroom must be individualized. CDC guidelines provide for periodic evaluation of infected individuals to monitor the progress of infection as well as assess the magnitude of risk presented. Increased risk may be presented, for example, by mental deterioration which produces uncontrolled behavior, or by the development of open sores which cannot be covered and present a significantly increased risk of exposure through otherwise casual contact. Some courts have been particularly sensitive to these policies and have incorporated them into the orders for admission for HIV infected students. However, repeated testing of an individual already known to be infected with HIV for the continued presence of HIV antibody serves no useful medical purpose, even though it has occasionally been ordered by courts as a part of the conditions for enrolling HIV infected students (*Ray* v. *School District of DeSoto County*).

The emphasis of individual courts and commentators varies, but it now appears that the general approach to enrollment of HIV infected students should be threefold:

1. HIV infected students should ordinarily be enrolled in the normal classroom setting because the classroom does not generally present an increased risk of transmission.
2. Periodic, individualized evaluation of infected children is necessary to assess changing disease status and properly monitor the risk of transmission, as well as to properly provide for the care of the infected child.
3. Confidentiality of the infected student must be respected.

PRESUMPTIVE ENROLLMENT OF HIV INFECTED STUDENTS

An increasing number of educational institutions at all levels are adopting policies which provide that HIV infected individuals are presumptively fit for normal classroom attendance. Generally, such policies also depend on voluntary disclosure and discourage mandatory testing. The American Academy of Pediatrics and the CDC both emphasize that routine screening of school-aged children for HIV infection is not appropriate. Older students in college and university programs, or vocational-technical institutions should also be considered presumptively fit for enrollment unless the classroom environment is such that a significant increase in the risk of transmission is presented by an HIV infected student, and that risk cannot be controlled by appropriate environmental policies.

Both the Rehabilitation Act and the Education for All Handicapped Children Act would seem to dictate that a policy of presumptive suitability for enrollment is not only sensible but also necessary. The situations in which infected individuals present an increased risk of transmission are relatively few: children who are incapable of controlling biting or body functions (especially in young children); extensive skin sores, or severe behavior problems which may include biting or other aggressive behavior. Residential schools which deal with emotionally disturbed students who are incapable of controlling impulsive behavior may be presented with an insoluble problem if sexual activity between students cannot be prevented. Although no case law exists on this point, such a situation may be appropriate for segregation of HIV infected residents from those not infected with the virus if sexual transmission cannot be otherwise prevented. On this unsettled point, competent legal advice is necessary, taking into account the individual situation and emerging law. It has been established that rehabilitative programs which prohibit drug use and sexual relations between adult patients cannot exclude individuals on the basis of HIV infection if anti-discrimination laws apply (*Doe* v. *Centinela Hospital*), but the application of this principle to residential schools in which such contact, although discouraged, necessarily occurs between individuals who are incapable of either understanding the risk of their actions or modifying their behavior, remains to be seen.

Other, accidental exposures, such as from bloody noses or accidental needlesticks, can, and should be, adequately controlled by general infection control policies designed to limit exposure to *any* foreign blood or body fluid. This is especially important since not all cases of HIV infection will be identified, even with an active screening program an unsuspected infection is just as capable of transmitting HIV infection as is known disease.

INDIVIDUALIZED EVALUATION

Once HIV infected students are identified, a multidisciplinary team, which includes the treating physician, public health authorities, teachers, administrators and the parents, is advisable to provide periodic assessment of the safety of the classroom environment for the infected student as well as others. Such a team may be a resource to the family, student and school for support and education to reduce the discrimination against and harassment of infected students. The wisest course is to address the possibility of enrolling HIV infected students before the issue actually arises, developing a team approach and defining community resources, so that when enrollment of the first student known to be infected with HIV occurs, it is handled as a matter of legally sound and well defined policy rather than as a crisis.

The ordinary classroom presents increased risk to the immunosuppressed child, whether this results from HIV infection, treatment for cancer, or other underlying diseases. Epidemic infections such as chicken pox, which are common in schools, are potentially devastating to students with poorly functioning immune systems. A properly constructed supervisory team can also alert the treating physician of immunosuppressed children of infectious risks to the HIV infected student, allowing for proper prophylaxis and treatment. Alternative education plans, such as for home schooling, should also be provided until the risk is passed. Because it is not possible to know with certainty which students are HIV infected or otherwise immune suppressed, information about the presence of epidemic illness such as meningitis or chickenpox within the school should be made available to all students and their families.

CONFIDENTIALITY

In order best to serve the needs of the HIV infected student, some key personnel will be aware of the diagnosis. However, it is imperative that information about HIV infection be treated with the strictest confidence, and limited to those who legitimately need to know in order to adequately protect the infected student as well as his peers. School records should not be flagged with conspicuous markers indicating HIV infection, whether educational records or medical records. School personnel should be made aware of the risks of improper communication of any information about students. Hallway consultations, indiscreet conversations and poor control of private records, whether or not related to HIV infection, expose the school to liability for breach of confidence, and should be avoided.

Because it is advisable to implement general infection control policies, fewer individuals have a legitimate claim to knowledge about a student's HIV status. Publication of a clear cut policy about who will, and will not, be informed, as well as statements of confidentiality, will help limit claims of concealment and decrease unrealistic expectations. It also serves to alert students, faculty and staff of their own personal responsibility to adhere to reasonable standards of hygiene and personal conduct. Students, parents, faculty and staff should be told in no uncertain terms that information about HIV infection of students is a private matter that cannot and will not be disclosed under school policies, and is not permitted by law. In concert with such a policy, access to educational programs, materials and resource persons should be encouraged. Not only must the school make it clear that infection is unlikely as a result of school contact, it must be emphasized again and again that personal habits offer the only reasonable hope of avoiding infection, inside or outside the school. Beginning to encourage the development of sound personal habits in students, and emphasizing that the parents must play a substantial role in the development of such habits should be a top priority.

If the school is aware of a student who is HIV infected and is, by his habits, exposing others to infection by, for example, unprotected intercourse or drug abuse, the issue of a duty to warn must be addressed. The current trend of protecting confidentiality suggests that only in the most extreme situations would a duty arise with respect to the school. No blanket recommendations can be made on this point because each case is individual in the balance of personal and societal rights. Competent legal assistance should be sought. Referring the matter to public health officials for action under their statutory powers is one possibility which should not be overlooked. Schools should also exercise every effort to insure that lax enforcement of policies about drug abuse on campus do not afford opportunities for transmission of HIV infection that would not otherwise exist on campus. It should also be kept in mind that violation of rules concerning drug use, cohabitation or any other legitimate institutional rules, if applied evenly to all students and if implemented with proper regard for due process, may offer a means to remove a student from the environment regardless of HIV infection.

RESIDENCE HALL POLICIES

Studies which confirm the lack of transmission of HIV among household contacts indicate that residence halls should present relatively little risk for HIV transmission. However, intimate contact which is potentially capable of transmitting infection, such as sharing personal articles such as razors, toothbrushes and other items which may carry traces of blood and which should not be shared with an individual who is infected with HIV, according to medical guidelines, is more likely in the residence hall than in the classroom. Whether to isolate HIV infected students, and when to notify roommates are common concerns. Some institutions provide single rooms for HIV infected students. Such a policy is probably acceptable if:

(1) it is not limited only to HIV infected students, because this could be construed as discrimination in light of the fact that other diseases present a much greater risk of transmission;

(2) it does not cost the student more, because both the Rehabilitation Act and EAHCA require the costs of accommodation be borne by the institution and not the individual; and

(3) it is not mandatory, because mandatory isolation in the absence of medical indications, is almost certainly discriminatory.

The American College Health Association recommends that no special provisions be made unless medically indicated or requested by the student. Notification of the roommate is almost certainly prohibited unless authorized by the student or if the roommate is definitely at risk because of sexual contact or drug abuse. Even then, it is questionable whether notification of the roommate is permissible given the great emphasis on the confidentiality of HIV related information that is emerging under current laws. On the balance, the most prudent procedure for managing residence halls would seem to include:

(1) a well publicized policy of confidentiality, making students aware that they may be assigned a roommate who is infected with HIV and, if so, will not be informed by the school;

(2) AIDS education as a part of student orientation, including the distribution of student handbooks containing information, and the establishment of resources which are available to students who desire counseling, testing or more information;

(3) accommodation of HIV infected students who because of their medical condition require either private rooms or live-in assistance;

(4) a confidential residence hall committee to which students may disclose HIV infection, or discuss other HIV related concerns, and who will facilitate accommodation of the student. Residence halls offer an especially effective forum for AIDS education. Proper training of residence hall associates and identification of community resources available to respond to student questions and needs, are essential.

AIDS EDUCATION

The constraints of discrimination and privacy law prevent notification of HIV infection, absent consent of the infected individual, in nearly all casual settings. Such settings may still be the forum in which HIV infection is acquired because of high risk behavior or lack of understanding about the transmission of the disease. Control of HIV infection is, and will remain, largely behavioral: avoid risky situations and one avoids the disease. Consequently, considerable effort should be directed at programs which educate students, faculty and staff about the biology of HIV infection, how to avoid infection, and how to identify high risk behavior.

Educational programs should include age appropriate sex and drug information, but should also emphasize the proper handling of blood and body fluids. In the school environment, this is particularly important because the popularly perceived risks of transmission from exposure to blood can be controlled through properly implemented disinfection policies coupled with sound educational programs.

The personal and emotional toll of HIV infection should not be neglected in an educational program. Some emphasis should be given activities which are *safe:* sharing a common classroom or office, touching, shaking hands, sharing toilet facilities, showers, pools or eating facilities. The great majority of human activity is without risk with respect to HIV transmission, yet many HIV infected individuals are completely shunned and isolated. Compassionate explanation of the few activities which are potentially risky and an emphasis on the need of HIV infected individuals to remain among their peers may help reduce the negative responses of associates. Preventive education and programs directed at reintegrating infected persons within the classroom or office setting are critical to the success of any educational program.

Education is particularly important for health care workers and students, because the risk of significant exposure is markedly increased. Copies of appropriate infection control policies should be routinely provided to students and staff in health care programs. Some institutions also require a signed statement of receipt, reading and understanding of the policies, which is highly recommended as proof that the institution has fulfilled its duty of notification and education with respect to HIV infection control policies. Proper education of health professionals and students in health care related programs is an essential in any health care training program. Even if practical training is taken outside the institution, it is incumbent upon the school to provide adequate training in proper health and safety procedures, including HIV infection control. This is a duty of the school in which the student is enrolled and cannot be delegated safely to other institutions.

Because AIDS education requires discussing sex in a frank and open manner, administrators should anticipate that some parents will object to their children being exposed to information about HIV infection and transmission. Ultimately, some of these children will have to be excused from participation on the same basis that some children are excused from more conventional sex-education programs. However, given the importance of AIDS education, it is probably prudent that school officials faced with excusing students on the basis of parental objections meet with the objecting parents individually, in the company of public health officials, if possible, in an effort to emphasize the need to participate. If the parents remain unconvinced, it should be documented in writing, signed by the parent, that the school attempted to inform the parent of the importance of AIDS education, and that the failure of the child to participate could deprive the child of life-saving information. "Watered down" education which fails to address the pertinent sexual and social aspects of HIV transmission is not desirable, but may be held in reserve to offer to students whose parents simply cannot or will not permit otherwise adequate education of their children, on the theory that any education about AIDS is better than total ignorance.

HIV STATUS AND PARTICIPATION IN PARTICULAR PROGRAMS

Administrators mindful of the costs of academic programs, particularly athletic scholarship programs, often inquire whether HIV screening can be incorporated as part of the required physical examination for participation in school programs. If HIV infection can be shown to be a legitimate disqualification because it renders an individual incapable of fully participating in the program, the testing may legitimately be done. In most programs, however, including sports programs, HIV infection alone has no effect on the ability of the student to participate. Thus, for all intents and purposes, schools cannot seek HIV information under the guise of a required physical exam, and then use the information for discriminatory purposes.

HIV infection alone is not sufficiently predictive of future illness, either in time or degree, to limit student participation in athletic programs. The fear of HIV transmission because of bleeding injuries commonly sustained in contact sports has been cited as a reason to require HIV testing of student athletes. The risk of transmission, even in these situations is low and can be adequately handled by appropriate universal precautions limiting all exposure to blood and body fluids. For these reasons, HIV testing of athletes is generally not supportable. Nor may they be tested on the theory that HIV infection predisposes to future incapacity, since qualifications for team participation, enrollment and scholarship purposes must be determined in the present rather than the future.

Students in the health professions should be offered the opportunity to be tested for HIV infection. Because the CDC currently recognizes no positions from which a health professional should be barred, if HIV infected, for fear of transmission to patients, exclusion from training programs on this basis is not justified. Exclusion of symptomatic individuals because of the inability to participate in a rigorous training program may be justified but must be well supported by sound medical evidence. Any action to limit the participation of HIV infected students in such circumstances must be undertaken cautiously and only on advice of counsel, because it clearly goes against the general norm mandating participation of HIV infected students in most academic programs.

Students who elect to participate in foreign study may be appropriately screened for HIV infection, if the fact of infection would prohibit their entry into a foreign nation, or, possibly, if they will be sent to remote areas in which no proper medical facilities are available for treatment if infection becomes symptomatic. If inability to obtain appropriate visas is at issue, screening need not be done by the school, which has only to require that the appropriate visa be obtained. If exclusion is contemplated on medical grounds, however, the concerned officials must be aware that it is possible, if not likely, that courts will consider the policy to be paternalistic and discriminatory, and therefore impermissible. At the present time, HIV screening of foreign study students is not recommended.

More important than screening foreign study students is the duty of schools sponsoring foreign study programs to be certain that participating students are aware of the risks of participating. This may include exposure to infectious diseases, including AIDS. The limited health care facilities in certain parts of the world, as well as the contamination of blood supplies are important information that students and their parents must be aware of in order to make a responsible decision about participation in foreign study. In some parts of the world, for example, the blood supply is so contaminated with HIV that surgery requiring blood transfusion may carry a 10 to 25% risk of contracting HIV infection. Caution dictates that such information be made readily available, especially to students who are likely to need medical care during their time abroad.

Chapter XI

Testing and Screening

AIDS is considered a handicap under the Rehabilitation Act of 1974. Silent HIV infection is also considered a protected handicap. Thus, the ability of an institution to screen for the presence of HIV infection is severely limited by the general proscriptions which prevent a school from actively seeking information about handicaps in its students rather than depending on elective disclosure by the student. The use of information about HIV infection from screening programs is severely limited by the dictates of the Rehabilitation Act, even when information is known about HIV infection. Any institution considering implementing a screening program for HIV infection must address several issues: the circumstances in which the test results may be used, the relationship of HIV infection to valid disability, and the adverse economic and social impact of implementing a screening program. The relative balance among these factors will determine whether HIV screening is a useful procedure.

In most instances, general screening will not be productive and in fact, will be detrimental to the institution attempting to implement it. Even if testing is carried out validly under a general physical examination, test results may not be used to discriminate against individuals in violation of the Rehabilitation Act and other, related anti-discrimination legislation. Further, in most cases, HIV infection itself is not a disability which prevents participation in the workplace or in academic programs. Rather than emphasizing screening for HIV, effort should be directed at detecting incapacity from any cause which may prevent full participation in school or work activity regardless of its cause.

The probability of future incapacity cannot generally be used as a basis for discrimination on the basis of a handicap protected under the Rehabilitation Act or related anti-discrimination laws. In the case of full-blown AIDS, the certainty of imminent death may justify the restriction of some positions requiring extensive or expensive training. However, silent HIV infection is not very predictive of ultimate incapacity, either in time or degree because of the great variability in clinical course and the long latent period. Thus, screening programs to seek silent HIV infection are probably not viable.

Mandatory screening of students is not recommended by the CDC, American Academy of Pediatrics, or the American College Health Association. If medically sound cause to suspect infection exists, however, such as known exposure or clinical symptoms, it may be appropriate to suggest appropriate medical attention, including testing for HIV infection.

If testing is done for any reason, it must be performed only by qualified laboratories capable of high quality work. Action taken on the basis of HIV infection must be supported by sound medical evidence, which includes confirmatory testing by Western Blot, or other state of the art means. No action against a student or employee should ever be taken on the basis of low specificity screening tests such as ELISA alone, nor should such results be reported to the individual as positive until properly confirmed.

It is incumbent on any institution which provides testing for HIV to insure that the demands of informed consent are met. This includes providing the individual to be tested, with information about the meaning of test results, the need for confirmation of screening tests, and appropriate information regarding the prevention of transmission of HIV infection, the desirability of testing contacts of HIV infected persons and the availability of public health services. Some states have adopted statutes which mandate specific informational and counseling requirements both before and after the test is drawn, and which also impose severe penalties for failure to comply with statutory procedures. Even absent statutory requirements, proper counseling is imperative whenever HIV testing is contemplated. If proper counseling and support cannot be offered immediately and directly to those who are to be tested, HIV testing should not be done.

Schools at all levels should seek to avoid implementing mandatory testing programs, because most will be impermissible under anti-discrimination laws. Mandatory testing programs may be valid for laboratory personnel who will work closely with large amounts of highly infective HIV containing material either in hospitals or academic research laboratories. Other individuals who may be exposed to HIV as a result of class or job exposure, such as medical and nursing students, laboratory technicians, and paramedics should be offered the opportunity of testing on enrollment or hiring and at regular intervals or when exposure actually occurs, in keeping with accepted infection control guidelines. Testing in such situations is largely to manage institutional liability for on the job infection, and probably cannot be mandated over the objections of the student or employee. Documented refusal of a student or employee to avail himself of HIV testing, offered because of exposure in the course of educational activities, should be available to the institution as a defense against the possibility of any suit later filed claiming infection as a result of contact within the school.

Colleges and universities will find students seeking testing and counseling through their college health services. It is appropriate to offer testing services, as long as proper attention is paid to confidentiality and counseling. Referral to public health officials for elective testing requested by the student and not ordered as part of medical care will significantly reduce the liability of the school for improper testing, failure to keep confidential sensitive information, and failure to provide proper counseling. Particularly for small schools with limited health care services, this option should be strongly considered.

Appendix I

Home Care Guidelines
For HIV Infected Persons

The CDC issued guidelines for screening blood donors in January of 1985. Contained within that report were also recommendations for HIV infected individuals to help prevent transmission of the disease. Subsequent policies drafted by other health agencies and institutions have incorporated these and are briefly summarized below:

1. HIV infection is lifelong. Even if asymptomatic, infection may be transmitted to others by anal sex, vaginal sex and sharing of needles. Oral-genital contact and deep kissing may also transmit the infection and should be avoided.

2. Use of condoms may reduce transmission of the virus but do not completely eliminate the risk.

3. Any implement which may become contaminated with blood should not be shared unless properly disinfected. This includes personal items such as thermometers, razors, scissors, tweezers, and toothbrushes. If the HIV infected individual has bleeding gums or diarrhea, separate tableware should be used. Separate bottles and nipples should be reserved for infants with HIV infection.

4. Gloves should be worn when handling soiled linen, bandages and any other material contaminated by blood, urine, feces, vomitus or other body fluids. Frequent handwashing and good general hygiene is encouraged.

5. Disinfection should be done with a 1:10 solution of household bleach in water.

6. Hot water washing with added Lysol® and/or bleach is recommended for clothing and linens.

7. Waste should be double-bagged in impermeable plastic, secured with twist ties and discarded.

For additional information see:

CDC, Provisional PHS interagency recommendations for screening donated blood and plasma for antibody to the virus causing immunodeficiency syndrome, 34 MMWR 1 (1985)

Magallon, Counseling patients with HIV infections, ___ Medical Aspects of Human Sexuality, 129 (June, 1987)

Lang, *et. al.* Living with AIDS: A Self Care Manual, AIDS Project Los Angeles (1986)

Keeling, AIDS on the College Campus: ACHA Special Report, American College Health Association (1986)

Appendix II

Guidelines for Infection Control Issued by CDC

Space does not permit reproducing all current Center for Disease Control (CDC) guidelines with respect to AIDS. The following is a list of individual CDC Recommendations and Policies regarding various aspects of AIDS transmission, treatment and diagnosis. Recently, a summary volume containing the most commonly requested and utilized guidelines has also become available.

Education and foster care of children infected with HTLV-III/LAV, 34 MMWR 517 (1985)

Recommendations for prevention of HIV transmission in health care settings, 36 MMWR 2S (1987)

CDC Guidelines on AIDS in the Workplace (Recommendations for preventing transmission of infection with HTLV-III/LAV in the workplace), 34 MMWR __ (November 14, 1985)

AIDS precautions for health care workers and allied professionals, 32 MMWR 450 (1983) (includes morticians and dentists)

Recommendations for preventing transmission of infection with human T-lymphotrophic virus type III-lymphadenopathy associated virus during invasive procedures, 35 MMWR 221 (1986)

Recommendations for assisting in the prevention of perinatal transmission of human T-lymphotrophic virus type III-lymphadenopathy associated virus and AIDS, 34 MMWR 721 (1985)

Additional recommendations to reduce sexual and drug abuse related transmission of human T-lymphotrophic virus type III-lymphadenopathy associated virus, 35 MMWR 152 (1986)

Immunizing children infected with human T-lymphotrophic virus type III-lymphadenopathy associated virus, 34 MMWR 231 (1986)

Safety of therapeutic immune globulin preparations with respect to human T-lymphotrophic virus type III-lymphadenopathy associated virus, 34 MMWR 231 (1986)

Recommended infection control practices for dentistry, 35 MMWR 237 (1986)

Recommendations for preventing possible transmission of human T-lymphotrophic virus type III-lymphadenopathy associated virus from tears, 34 MMWR 533 (1985)

Recommendations for providing dialysis treatment to patients infected with human T-lymphotrophic virus type III-lymphadenopathy associated virus, 35 MMWR 376 (1986)

Diagnosis and management of mycobacterial infection and disease in persons with human T-lymphotrophic virus type III-lymphadenopathy associated virus infection, 35 MMWR 448 (1986)

Appendix III

Guidelines and Procedures Concerning HIV, ARC, and AIDS*

Dated September 1, 1987

INTRODUCTION

Epidemiologic studies show that HIV is transmitted via contact with the body fluids of an infected person. Since there is no evidence of casual transmission by sitting near, living in the same household, or playing together with an individual who has HIV infection, the following guidelines have been developed with the guidance of members of the medical community for the School Board of Sarasota County, Florida:

I. **Student Guidelines and Procedures**

    A. All children diagnosed as having HIV, ARC or AIDS including clinical evidence of infection with the AIDS-associated virus (HIV) and receiving medical attention are able to attend regular classes. However, if a child so diagnosed evidences any one of the following conditions, the Superintendent of Schools will convene an Advisory Panel for the purpose of making recommendations on the most appropriate educational placement of the student:

        1. Manifestation of clinical signs and/or symptoms which indicate progression of illness from *Covert* (HIV infection only) to *Overt* status (ARC or AIDS Related Complex) or from *Overt* status to *Disability* (AIDS or Acquired Immune Deficiency Syndrome) or from *Disability* to *Debilitation* (late stage disease).

        2. Demonstration of risky or harmful behavior to self or others.

        3. Unstable or decompensated neuropsychological behavior.

---

*Reprinted with permission of The School Board of Sarasota County, Florida.

4. Presence of open wounds, cuts, lacerations, abrasions, or sores on exposed body surfaces where occlusion cannot be maintained.
5. Impairment of gastro-intestinal and/or genito-urinary function such that control of internal body fluids cannot be maintained.

B. *Composition of the Advisory Panel:*
1. Superintendent of the School Board of Sarasota County.
2. Director and Health Officer of Sarasota County Health Department.
3. Attending physician of the person with HIV infection.
4. Secretary to the Superintendent, to serve ex-officio as official recorder of the panel's review meeting.
5. Parent(s) of the HIV-infected student, when and as appropriate or requested.
6. Infectious disease specialty physician, when and as determined by the Superintendent as appropriate.
7. Legal counsel for School Board, when and as determined by the Superintendent as appropriate.
8. Legal counsel of HIV-infected person, when and as appropriate or requested.
9. Other school district staff including SC/TA representation, when and as appropriate.

Persons listed in numbers 1-4 shall constitute the Advisory Panel. Persons listed in numbers 5-8 (and others when requested) may participate at the invitation of the Superintendent or at their request.

C. *Panel Responsibilities:*
1. Review student's medical history and current status.
2. Review available educational and social data, progress reports as available, test results, prior school placements, etc.
3. Advise parents of educational options, if applicable.
4. Assess risk-benefit options; then present and discuss options of home education, special education, other choices with parents/student, if applicable.
5. Reduce findings, options, and recommendations to writing and review draft report before submission to Superintendent, focusing on key issues, unresolved problems if any, and summary recommendations.
6. Submit written report to Superintendent and remain available as needed.
7. Re-evaluate all Panel cases on a continuing basis at least once every six months and more often as circumstances change in the categories listed in *A* above.

The general intent of the Advisory Panel is to serve as an expert professional resource to advise the Superintendent in special situations where information about appropriate environment may not be available, complete, clear, or readily amenable to lay interpretation. It is expected that recommendations of the Advisory Panel shall be based solely upon current medical and educational information consistent with established ethical guidelines and considerations in accordance with extant Guidelines of the Centers for Disease Control and other scientific and relevant professional bodies.

D. *Panel Protocol:*

1. If the Superintendent determines that any one of the conditions in *A* exists, the student in question will be placed on homebound instruction status for no longer than five school days.

2. Within the five school day period (equivalent to one calendar week), consent for release of medical information will be obtained and past medical history, laboratory tests, and other relevant records will be provided to and reviewed by the Director of the Health Department and other physicians as appropriate. Critical medical tests and other procedures will be conducted during this period by the Director of the Health Department or other Medical practitioners as warranted.

3. Based on results and medical interpretation of the person's current status, the Director of the Health Department (and other consultants as appropriate) will advise the Superintendent within five days if continued home instruction is or is not warranted.

4. If medical review indicates that continuation of special status is not indicated, the student will return to regular status at the end of the five school day initial review period or upon the advice of the Director of the Health Department, whichever is sooner.

5. If medical review indicates that continuation of special status is indicated, the student will remain on home instruction, for a period not to exceed fifteen additional school days (or three more calendar weeks).

6. During the twenty school day review period, the Superintendent will arrange the following steps in preparation for Advisory Panel review:

   a. Alert Advisory Panel of forthcoming meeting to be scheduled.

b. Obtain written authorization from parents of student to contact attending physician for medical information.

c. Obtain signed consent from parent(s) of student to permit release of information from attending physician and others to Superintendent of Sarasota County Public Schools.

d. Receive relevant medical and social information about the person with HIV infection and maintain same in strict confidence.

e. Circulate confidential information about the HIV-infected person to Advisory Panel members only.

f. Schedule and notify Advisory Panel members of initial review meeting, at date, time and location suitable to all. (To be set up only when complete medical information has been obtained and circulated in advance to all Advisory Panelists).

E. Siblings of children diagnosed as having HIV, ARC, AIDS or with clinical evidence of infection with the AIDS-associated virus (HIV) are able to attend school without any restrictions.

F. Only persons with an absolute need to know should have medical knowledge of a particular student's case. In individual situations, the Superintendent may notify one or more of the following: 1) Principal; 2) School Nurse; 3) Student's Teacher. Notification should be made through a process that would maximally ensure patient confidentiality. Ideally, this process should be direct person-to-person contact. Persons who become so informed will be expected to maintain strict confidentiality.

G. Since the student diagnosed as having clinical evidence of infection with the AIDS-associated virus (HIV, ARC or AIDS) has an increased risk of acquiring infections in the school setting, the student will be excluded from school if there is an outbreak of a threatening communicable disease such as chicken pox or measles, until he/she is properly treated (possibly with hyperimmune gamma globulin) and/or the outbreak is no longer a threat to the child.

H. Blood or any other body fluids including vomitus and fecal or urinary products of *any* student should be treated cautiously. It is required that gloves be worn when cleaning up any body fluids from any student.

1. These spills should be cleaned up with a fresh solution of bleach (no older than 24 hours; one part bleach to ten parts water) or another EPA and District approved disinfectant, by pouring the solution around the perimeter of the spill.

2. All disposable materials, including gloves, should be discarded in a plastic bag. The mop should also be disinfected with the bleach solution described above.
3. Persons involved in the clean-up should wash their hands afterwards with soap.
I. In-service programs for all staff will be conducted as required and as new information becomes available.

II. Employee Guidelines and Procedures

A. *Statement of Purpose and Scope*

This section establishes the policy of the School Board of Sarasota county, Florida for working with employees who have HIV, ARC or AIDS. Its purpose is the protection of the right of such school district's employees to continued employment. The school board recognizes its obligation as an employer to provide not only an objectively safe environment for all employees and the public at large, but also an environment where employees and students do not have fears for their health and safety.

The policy and procedures are applicable to all employees of the School Board of Sarasota County, Florida.

B. *Employee Policy*

The school board recognizes that employees with life-threatening illnesses, including, but not limited to, cancer, heart disease, and AIDS related illnesses may wish to continue to work. As long as employees are able to meet acceptable performance standards, and medical evidence indicates that their condition is not a threat to themselves or others, employees shall be assured of continued employment. Federal and State laws also mandate, pursuant to the laws protecting disabled individuals, that those individuals not be discriminated against on the basis of their handicaps, and that if it becomes necessary, some reasonable accommodations be made to enable qualified individuals to continue to work.

C. *Training and Education*

Medical studies show that HIV infection (which can lead to AIDS) is transmitted via contact with body fluids of an infected person. To date, there is no record of transmission of the AIDS associated virus (HIV) to co-workers, clients or consumers in offices, schools, factories, construction sites or other workplaces. There is no evidence of casual transmission by sitting near, working in the same office, sharing the same water fountain, telephones, toilets, eating facilities or office equipment with a person infected with HIV.

Many of the problems which arise in the workplace when employees are confronted with a fellow employee who has become HIV infected are caused by lack of knowledge about the disease and misunderstanding of the ways in which it is transmitted. The only means of combatting this fear is education. Supervisors should make a concerted effort to educate themselves as to the facts regarding HIV infection and how it is and is not transmitted and, further, should make the same effort to educate their employees. Any information needed will be furnished by the Division of Instruction. Supervisors should be sensitive and responsive to co-workers' concerns, and emphasize employee education.

D. *Confidentiality*

The School Board realizes that an employee's health condition is personal and confidential. Personnel and medical files or information about employees are exempt from public disclosure. In addition, information relating to a specifically-named individual, the disclosure of which would constitute an unwarranted invasion of personal privacy is prohibited. Thus, special precautions should be taken to protect such information regarding an employee's health condition in order to prevent instances of disclosure that may invade the personal privacy of employees. Only those supervisors with a clear need to know should be informed of an employee's health condition.

E. Any staff member diagnosed as having HIV, ARC or AIDS, (including clinical evidence of infection with the AIDS-associated virus (HIV)) and receiving medical attention is not prohibited from reporting for duty. However, if an employee so diagnosed evidences any of the following conditions, the Superintendent of Schools may convene an Advisory Panel for the purpose of making recommendations on the most appropriate work assignment for the employee:

1. Manifestation of clinical signs and/or symptoms which indicate progression of illness from *Covert* (HIV infection only) to *Overt* status (ARC or AIDS Related Complex) or from *Overt* status to *Disability* (AIDS or Acquired Immune Deficiency Syndrome) or from *Disability* to *Debilitation* (late stage disease).
2. Demonstration of risky or harmful behavior to self or others.
3. Unstable or decompensated neuropsychological behavior.
4. Presence of open wounds, cuts, lacerations, abrasions, or sores on exposed body surfaces where occlusion cannot be maintained.

5. Impairment of gastro-intestinal and/or genito-urinary function such that control of internal body fluids cannot be maintained.

F. *Composition of the Advisory Panel:*
1. Superintendent of the School Board of Sarasota County.
2. Director and Health Officer of Sarasota County Health Department.
3. Attending physician of the employee with HIV infection.
4. Secretary to the Superintendent, to serve ex-officio as official recorder of the panel's review meeting.
5. Infectious disease specialty physician, when and as determined by the Superintendent as appropriate.
6. Legal counsel for School Board, when and as determined by the Superintendent as appropriate.
7. Legal counsel, union representative or other advisor of the employee, when and as appropriate or requested.
8. Other school district staff, when and as appropriate.

Persons listed in numbers 1-4 shall constitute the Advisory Panel. Persons listed in numbers 5-8 (and others when requested) may participate at the invitation of the Superintendent or at their request.

G. *Panel Responsibilities:*
1. Review employee's medical history and current status.
2. Review available social data, prior school assignments, employment history, etc.
4. Assess risk-benefit options; then present and discuss employment options with employee, if applicable.
5. Reduce findings, options, and recommendations to writing and review draft report before submission to Superintendent, focusing on key issues, unresolved problems if any, and summary recommendations.
6. Submit written report to Superintendent and remain available as needed.
7. Re-evaluate all Panel cases on a continuing basis at least once every six months and more often as circumstances change in the categories listed in *E* above.

The general intent of the Advisory Panel is to serve as an expert professional resource to advise the Superintendent in special situations where information about appropriate environment may not be available, complete, clear, or readily amenable to lay interpretation. It is expected that recommendations of the Advisory Panel shall be based solely upon current medical and employment information consistent with established ethical guidelines and considerations in accordance with extant Guidelines of the Centers for Disease Control and other scientific and relevant professional bodies.

H. *Panel Protocol:*

1. If the Superintendent determines that any one of the conditions in *E* exists, the employee in question will be placed on sick leave status for no longer than five work days.

2. Within the five work day period (equivalent to one calendar week), consent for release of medical information will be obtained and past medical history, laboratory tests, and other relevant records will be provided to and reviewed by the Director of the Health Department and other physicians as appropriate. Critical medical tests and other procedures will be conducted during this period by the Director of the Health Department or other medical practitioners as warranted.

3. Based on results and medical interpretation of the employee's current status, the Director of the Health Department (and other consultants as appropriate) will advise the Superintendent within five days if continued sick leave is or is not warranted.

4. If medical review indicates that continuation of special status is not indicated, the employee will return to regular status at the end of the five school day initial review period or upon the determination of the Superintendent, whichever is sooner.

5. If medical review indicates that continuation of special status is indicated, the employee will remain on sick leave or special assignment for a period not to exceed fifteen additional work days (or three more calendar weeks).

6. During the twenty school day review period, the Superintendent will arrange the following steps in preparation for Advisory Panel review:

   a. Alert Advisory Panel of forthcoming meeting to be scheduled.

   b. Obtain written authorization from employee to contact attending physician for medical information.

   c. Obtain signed consent from employee to permit release of information from attending physician and others to Superintendent of Sarasota County Public Schools.

   d. Receive relevant medical and social information about the employee with HIV infection and maintain same in strict confidence.

e. Circulate confidential information about the HIV-infected employee to Advisory Panel members only.
f. Schedule and notify Advisory Panel members of initial review meeting, at date, time and location suitable to all. (To be set up only when complete medical information has been obtained and circulated in advance to all Advisory Panelists).

Appendix IV

General Statement On Institutional Response to AIDS*

Revised November 1988

INTRODUCTION

The American College Health Association (ACHA) presents these recommendations and guidelines for institutions of higher education in response to the epidemic of infection with Human Immunodeficiency Virus (HIV), which causes the Acquired Immune Deficiency Syndrome (AIDS). This statement updates the editions of the *General Statement on Institutional Response to AIDS* issued December 2, 1985, and January 1, 1988. The recommendations and guidelines herein are based on the best currently available medical information and on statements by the United States Public Health Service and the Centers for Disease Control. ACHA has released detailed information and guidelines in certain specific areas of concern to colleges and universities in a special report, *AIDS on the College Campus.* Periodic future statements will update the special report and address other issues as they arise.

Communities in higher education must respond effectively to the epidemic of HIV infection. In a campus environment many students encounter new independence, self determination, and strong peer pressure to adopt certain behaviors. For some students, an uncertain sense of identity and self-esteem can further complicate decision-making. Experimentation with sexual behaviors and/or drug use may put college and university students at a greater risk of infection. Young adults often feel invincible and tend to deny personal risk. Many people in campus communities believe that HIV infection and AIDS are problems faced elsewhere, or are concerns only for "other kinds" of people. The prolonged latency between infection with HIV and the eventual development of full-blown AIDS will promote the relative invisibility of the infection, an effect that will seem to validate the myth

---

*Reprinted with permission of The American College Health Association from *AIDS on the College Campus,* second edition (1989).

97

among students (and some faculty and administrators) that "it cannot happen here."

HIV infection is potentially lethal, but absolutely preventable. Each college or university community must do more than be aware of the risks of HIV infection. Each community must accept that HIV infection and AIDS can, in fact, happen on any campus. Every institution of higher education must be accountable to its community to do everything possible to prevent people from being infected, to limit the consequences of established infection, and to provide compassionate care for all concerned individuals. These challenges will demand strong leadership and commitment.

ACHA acknowledges the valuable assistance of the American Council on Education (ACE) in the development of guidelines pertaining to the legal issues and questions presented by the epidemic of HIV infection, and appreciates the support of the National Association of Student Personnel Administrators and the Association of College and University Housing Officers-International.

EDUCATIONAL PROGRAMS

The primary response of colleges and universities to the epidemic of HIV infection must be education. The American College Health Association recommends that the organization and implementation of effective educational programs about AIDS and HIV infection be an activity of the highest priority for all institutions of higher learning. In designing the format and content of educational programs, it is important to recognize and address the rich diversity of people in the campus community and to provide opportunities for effective learning by people of any age, ability, gender, ethnicity, or sexual orientation.

Because there is as yet neither a vaccine to prevent HIV infection nor curative therapy for persons infected with HIV, the most pressing need for institutions will be to implement programs that increase awareness and provide education to prevent further spread of the virus. Although knowledge about limiting the consequences of established HIV infection is only beginning to develop, it is important that AIDS education programs also provide what information is available. The following are specific recommendations concerning educational programs:

1. Comprehensive educational programs must address not only undergraduates, but also graduate and professional students; they should reach not only residential students, but also commuters and non-traditional students. Programs to educate students about HIV infection and AIDS should also be available in junior and community colleges and in all schools offering post-secondary education, including continuing education programs.

2. Colleges and universities should offer similar educational opportunities for institutional employees, faculty, and staff. Providing education to faculty and other employees will require leadership from campus health and personnel officers and commitment from senior administrators.

3. The epidemic of HIV infection raises issues of liability that are of great concern to college and university administrators; currently the most effective means of addressing these issues is to educate students and employees about HIV infection and AIDS and to take such reasonable precautions as are suggested herein. Educational programs will also be of paramount importance in discharging the institution's responsibility to protect its student body and staff from the transmission of HIV. As medical evidence consistently indicates that no actual safety risks are created in the usual workplace or academic setting, institutions can best render enrollment or employment safe and healthful through effective education and training programs.

4. **The program of education provided by the institution should emphasize the following:**

a. Even though they may not have symptoms, persons with HIV infection may transmit the virus to others through intimate sexual contact or exposure to blood; a woman with HIV infection may transmit the virus to her child before or during birth or by breast feeding.

b. Among people who choose to be sexually active, the consistent and conscientious use of condoms and spermicides containing nonoxynol-9 greatly reduces the chance of transmission of HIV through sexual intercourse.

c. The sharing of needles used in the injection of illicit drugs is an efficient way to transmit HIV. It is possible that sharing needles used to inject steroids or for other reasons may transmit HIV as well.

d. Persons with documented HIV infection and those with behavioral risk factors for HIV infection should not donate blood, plasma, sperm, or other body organs or tissues.

e. People with HIV infection pose no risk of transmitting the virus to others through ordinary, casual interpersonal contact.

f. It is possible that certain interventions and therapies may help limit the consequences of HIV infection among people already infected. People who know they have been infected may thus benefit from regular medical follow-up and immunological evaluation.

g. Discrimination against people who have or are perceived to have HIV infection is unwarranted, hurtful, and wrong.

5. In colleges and universities with resident students, residence hall staff (both students and employees) should receive education about HIV infection and AIDS prior to the arrival of new students each session.

6. Students should play a major role in designing, implementing, and evaluating educational programs. Peer education models will be especially effective.

7. As a component of its educational program, an institution should inform students and employees about condoms and spermicides and their proper utilization. Condoms and spermicides should be readily available to all students. Colleges and universities may best accomplish this by vending condoms and spermicides in machines, which allows individuals to obtain these materials anonymously and outside regular business hours. Less effective alternatives to condom vending include distributing or selling condoms and spermicides in the health service or at campus stores and referring students to private retailers.

8. **In order for educational programs to be effective, they must provide current information, use reliable, up-to-date materials, and be both easily accessible and widely available.** The Task Force on AIDS of the American College Health Association produces and periodically updates educational brochures and videotapes dealing with various aspects of HIV infection and AIDS which are available to all institutions. Detailed recommendations for educational programs, including suggested formats and methodologies, are included in the special report, *AIDS on the College Campus.* ACHA will continue to release new educational materials, reports, and programming suggestions.

RECOMMENDED POLICIES

A. Application

These guidelines, which derive from the best currently available medical facts about HIV infection and AIDS, apply to all students or employees with HIV infection. People with HIV infection may be healthy, but have evidence of the infection because of the presence of an antibody to the virus in their blood; others have a condition meeting the criteria of the surveillance definition of AIDS itself, or one of the lesser symptomatic manifestations of infection (such as AIDS-related complex or progressive generalized lymphadenopathy).

B. Transmission Information Relative to Policies

Current knowledge indicates that students or employees with any form of HIV infection do not pose a health risk to other students or employees in an academic setting. HIV is transmitted perinatally, by intimate sexual contact, and by exposure to contaminated blood. Although HIV may be found in many body fluids and secretions of people who are infected, its presence is clearly correlated with transmission only in blood, semen, and female genital secretions; breast milk may transmit the virus to a nursing infant. There has been no confirmed case of transmission of HIV by any household, school, or other casual contact. The Public Health Service states that there is No Risk

100

created by living in the same place as an infected person, eating food handled by an infected person, being coughed or sneezed upon by an infected person, casual kissing, or swimming in a pool with an infected person. See the following statements:

Centers for Disease Control. Education and Foster Care of Children Infected with Human T-Lymphotropic Virus Type III/Lymphadenopathy-Associated Virus. *Morbidity and Mortality Weekly Report* 1985; 34:517-521.

Centers for Disease Control. Recommendations for Prevention of Transmission of Infection with Human T-Lymphotropic Virus Type III/Lymphadenopathy-Associated Virus in the Workplace, *Morbidity and Mortality Weekly Report* 1985; 34:681-6, 691-6.

Health care workers with clinical responsibilities and certain laboratory technicians have a very small but real risk of HIV infection through direct contact with contaminated blood or laboratory preparations. Most such exposures can be prevented by consistent adherence to established infection control guidelines.

These facts are the basis for the following guidelines.

C. Guidelines for Institutional Policy

1. General policies. The American College Health Association recommends that institutions adopt only general policies, such as are included herein, concerning students or employees with HIV infection. ACHA suggests that institutions respond to each case as required by its particular facts. Given the uncertain legal obligations and challenges involved, institutions are advised neither to devise nor to implement inflexible policies.

2. Institutional committee. It is appropriate for college and university officials to designate a group of administrators and faculty to manage the process of evaluating individual cases, to organize and oversee the educational program, and to provide a mechanism for making such policy decisions as become necessary.

3. Handicapping conditions. It is clear that persons with AIDS itself (and, possibly, those with other manifestations of HIV infection) will be considered as having handicapping conditions; in making decisions, college and university officers are advised to guarantee the legal rights of these individuals. Existing support services for people with handicapping conditions can be appropriately and effectively utilized by students or employees disabled by HIV infection.

4. Admissions. No institution of higher education should include consideration of the existence of any form of HIV infection in the initial admissions decision for people applying to attend the institution. The exclusion of people with HIV infection for reason of that infection constitutes unwarranted discrimination.

5. Attendance. College and university students who have HIV infection, whether they are symptomatic or not, should be allowed regular classroom attendance in an unrestricted manner as long as they are physically and mentally able to attend classes.

6. **Access to facilities.** There is no justification, medical or otherwise, for restricting the access of persons with HIV infection to student unions, theatres, restaurants, snack bars, gymnasiums, swimming pools, saunas, recreational facilities, or other common areas.

7. **Residential housing.** Decisions about housing for students with HIV infection must be made on a case-by-case basis. **The best currently available medical information does not indicate any risk to those sharing residence with infected individuals. There may, however, be reasonable concern in some circumstances for the health of students with immune deficiencies (of any origin) when those students might be exposed to certain contagious diseases (e.g. measles or chicken pox) in a close living situation.** Health officers and administrators in institutions with the flexibility to provide private rooms may wish to recommend that students with immune deficiencies be assigned private rooms in order to protect the health of the immunodeficient student— not to protect other students from them. The American College Health Association recognizes that the fear of HIV infection and AIDS may cause considerable pressure to be brought to bear on housing officers, and has provided a thorough discussion of options in residential housing in the special report, *AIDS on the College Campus.*

8. **Medical care.** The following recommendations pertain to the provision of clinical services to people with HIV infection.

   a. **Medical history.** Institutions of higher education should not routinely ask students to respond to questions about the existence of HIV infection. It is, however, appropriate in many institutions to encourage students with HIV infection to inform campus health care providers in order to enable the institution to provide them proper medical care, support, counsel, and education. This, like any other medical information, should be handled in a strictly confidential manner in accordance with the procedures and requirements in effect at the institution.

   b. **Medical and psychological follow-up.** Clinicians in health services and counseling centers should make provisions for medical, psychological, and support services that promote the best physical and mental health of persons with HIV infection. Institutions should organize these resources *prior* to their need to avoid causing anxiety and distress in individuals requiring assistance. If these services are beyond the scope of comparable services provided on campus, the institution should immediately identify other care providers who will see students by referral. The evolution of antiviral or immunomodulating therapies for HIV infection requires that campus health care providers be aware of current developments and practices in immunological evaluation and treatment. If these services are beyond the scope of patient care services offered on campus, health officers should be able to refer students or employees to other facilities.

c. **Contagious diseases.** Special precautions to protect the health of immunologically compromised individuals should be applied during periods of prevalence of certain casually contagious diseases, such as measles and chicken pox.

d. **Immunizations.** Persons known to have HIV infection should receive measles and rubella vaccination and need not be exempted from institutional requirements for those vaccinations. However, clinicians in health services should be aware of current recommendations for other immunizations in persons with HIV infection because of potentially serious consequences of their receiving live virus vaccines. Some vaccines required for foreign travel may be deleterious to the health of persons infected with HIV.

9. **HIV antibody testing.**

a. **Mandatory testing. College and university officials should not undertake programs of mandatory testing of either employees or students for antibody to HIV.** Mandatory testing programs will be cost-ineffective, counterproductive, and discriminatory.

b. **Voluntary.** College and university health services should be familiar with sources of testing for antibody to HIV, and should be able to refer students or employees requesting tests. Health care providers should understand the capabilities and limitations of the test, and should be able to counsel and educate persons who seek testing. Administrators and clinicians must be familiar with state and local laws and public health requirements regarding charting of results, release of confidential information, and reporting of test results.

Whether the tests are performed through the campus health service or not, they should be done if and ONLY if:

(1) **they can be anonymous or, if anonymous testing is not possible, strictly confidential**

(2) **Positive results on the screening test (ELISA test) are confirmed by another procedure, and**

(3) **both pre-test and post-test counseling are a mandated part of the program.**

10. **Confidentiality of information.** People known or suspected to have HIV infection, whether or not they have symptoms of illness have sometimes been victims of discrimination and physical or psychological abuse. The potential for discrimination and mistreatment of these individuals, and of persons thought to be at risk of infection, requires that confidential information concerning any aspect of HIV infection be handled with extraordinary care.

a. **Standards.** Guidelines concerning the handling of confidential material about people with HIV infection follow the general standards included in the American College Health Association's *Recommended Standards and Practices for a College Health Program,* fourth edition:

In general, it is recommended that no specific or detailed information concerning complaints or diagnosis be provided to faculty, administrators, or even parents, without the expressed written consent of the patient in each case. This position with respect to health record is supported by the Family Education Rights and Privacy Act of 1974.

b. **Release of information.** No person, group, agency, insurer, employer, or institution should be provided any medical information of any kind without the prior, written consent of the patient. **Given the possibility of the unintended or accidental compromise of the confidentiality of information, health officers should carefully weigh the importance of including any specific information about the existence of known HIV infection in the ordinary medical record except when circumstances of medical necessity mandate it. At minimum, the inclusion of any information regarding HIV infection in the medical record should be discussed with the patient prior to its entry.**

c. **Legal liability.** Health officials and other institutional officers must remember that all confidential medical information is protected by statutes and that any unauthorized disclosure of it may create legal liability. The duty of physicians and other health care providers to protect the confidentiality of information is superseded by the necessity to protect others only in very specific, life-threatening circumstances.

d. **"Need to know."** The number of people in the institution who are aware of the existence and/or identity of students or employees who have an HIV infection should be kept to an absolute minimum, both to protect the confidentiality and privacy of the infected persons and to avoid the generation of unnecessary fear and anxiety among other students and staff. ACHA has released a more detailed statement discussing the handling of confidential information as part of the special report, *AIDS on the College Campus.*

e. **Informing other students or employees.** There is absolutely no medical or other reason for institutions to advise students living in a residence hall of the presence there of students with HIV infection. Similarly, college and university officials should not reveal the identity of students or employees with HIV infection in any other setting. The responsibility to provide a safe living environment is best dealt with by educational programming, as discussed earlier. Sharing confidential information without consent may create liability and lead to harassment or discrimination.

f. **Public health reporting requirements.** College and university health services must strictly observe public health reporting requirements. In all jurisdictions, cases of AIDS meeting the criteria of the surveillance definition of the Centers for Disease Control must be reported to the local public health authorities. In a few areas, seropositivity for antibody to HIV is also reportable but must be kept confidential. The detailed revised surveillance definition for AIDS for case reporting purposes is included in:

Centers for Disease Control. Revision of the CDC Surveillance Case Definition for Acquired Immunodeficiency Syndrome. *Morbidity and Mortality Weekly Report* 1987; 36:1S.

g. **Secondary lists of records.** Neither health officers nor other administrators should keep lists or logs identifying individuals tested for antibody to HIV or known to be infected with HIV. The potential for compromise of confidential information far exceeds any conceivable benefit of such listings.

11. **Safety Precautions. All colleges and universities should adopt safety guidelines as proposed by the United States Public Health Service for the handling of the blood and body fluids of all persons, not just those previously known to have HIV infection.** These "universal precautions" are necessary because many people with HIV infection are not identified in advance. The same procedures should thus be followed for the handling of blood and body fluids of *any* student or employee.

a. **Disinfection.** Surfaces contaminated by blood or other body fluids can be successfully cleaned and disinfected with commercial disinfectant solutions or with household bleach, freshly diluted in a 1:10 solution.

b. **Health care providers.**

1. **Public Health Service procedures.** In order to prevent the accidental transmission of HIV in health care settings, institutions that operate health services, laboratories, or clinics for students or staff should implement current recommendations from the Public Health Service for infection control, and should monitor compliance with these procedures. Colleges and universities should provide educational programs about HIV infection and its transmission in health care settings to all clinical personnel. The following articles provide current recommendations.

Centers for Disease Control. Recommendations for Prevention of HIV Transmission in Health Care Settings. *Morbidity and Mortality Weekly Report* 1987; 36:2S.

Centers for Disease Control. Update: Universal Precautions for Prevention of Transmission of Human Immunodeficiency Virus, Hepatitis B Virus, and Other Bloodborne Pathogens in Health Care Settings. *Morbidity and Mortality Weekly Report* 1988; 37:377-382, 387-388.

Medical and nursing professionals, dentists and oral surgeons, dental hygienists, optometrists, other clinical service providers, and research laboratory technicians handling blood or body fluids should be familiar with recommended infection control‑procedures and should follow them consistently.

2. **Equipment.** College and university health services should use disposable, one-user needles and other equipment whenever such equipment will puncture the skin or mucous membranes of patients. The same safety precautions must be used with all patients. If disposable equipment is not available, any needles or other implements that puncture skin or mucous membranes should be steam sterilized by autoclave before re-use or safely discarded. Extreme caution should be exercised when handling sharp objects, particularly in disposing of needles.

c. **Teaching laboratories.** Colleges and universities should also adopt safety guidelines for the handling of blood and body fluids of all persons in teaching laboratories. Laboratory courses requiring exposure to blood, such as biology courses in which blood is obtained by finger prick for typing or examination, should use disposable equipment, and no lancets or other blood-letting devices should be re-used or shared. No students, except those in health care professions schools, should be required to obtain or process the blood of others.

12. **Support services.** The psychosocial consequences of actual or feared HIV infection are such that college and university students and employees may experience enough suffering to impair their health, interfere with academic or work performance, cause extreme psychological distress, disrupt plans, and cripple relationships. Psychological, emotional, and spiritual health may also be important allies for people with established HIV infection. **The American College Health Association therefore recommends that all institutions develop easily accessible and widely available support services through which concerned persons can receive counseling, assistance in locating and using social resources, and referrals for further assistance.** Often, these needs may be met through existing student services or employee assistance programs or by identifying community-based resources for referrals.

13. **Harassment.** As a result of the fear, anxiety, and anger that many people feel in reaction to AIDS, some students or employees who are either known to be or suspected of being infected with HIV may be subjected to either emotional or physical abuse, or both. Institutions of higher education should condemn all such occurrences as intolerable and respond to them quickly and effectively.

Forthcoming statements and reports from ACHA will address other educational and administrative issues as they arise.

Appendix V

Housing Policies*

J. Robert Wirag, H.S.D.
C. Arthur Sandeen, Ph.D.
Leonard S. Goldberg, Ph.D.

Institutions providing on-campus living have a duty to support a residential environment free of unreasonable risks. Typically, this duty is discharged through an administrative unit (e.g., Residence Life Program) that manages a safe and healthful living environment through facility maintenance, appropriate staffing, and sound programming. As facilitating resources for their institutions, residence life programs work with many other campus units—such as food services, athletics, financial aid, health service, counseling center, campus police, judicial affairs, academic affairs, minority student services, foreign student advisors, and public relations. Both collegial and programmatic cooperation are necessary if students' numerous academic, physical, emotional, spiritual, and social concerns are to be dealt with effectively. The inter-relationships of the complex medical, psychological, social, ethical, and legal issues involving HIV infection and AIDS demand smooth and consistent cooperation among these various campus offices.

Institutional officials must communicate and widely explain the housing policies and procedures concerning HIV infection and AIDS. The policies developed must be readily accessible, clearly presented, openly discussed, and comfortably understood at all levels of campus administration. They must receive consistent support within the institution—particularly by the residence life staff, from the resident assistants to the director. To do otherwise will undoubtedly result in confusion and may expose individuals or the institution to unreasonable risk and unnecessary liability.

As the number of cases of HIV infection and AIDS increases, it is likely that difficult decisions will confront greater numbers of housing

*Reprinted with permission of The American College Health Association from *AIDS on the College Campus,* second edition (1989).

officials. Residence life and housing administrators who have not yet had to deal with a student with AIDS, and AIDS-related illness, or a positive test for antibody to HIV cannot afford to ignore the issues they will have to face. Officers in every residential institution must undertake planning now to prepare for such an eventuality. Housing directors must consider "worst case" scenarios and "what if" exercises and agree with other campus officials on measures to effectively man-

---

The policies developed must be readily accessible,
clearly presented, openly discussed,
and comfortably understood
at all levels of campus administration.

---

age decisions that will affect (1) students with AIDS, and AIDS-related illness, or a positive test for antibody to HIV, (2) other students concerned with AIDS-related issues, or (3) the interests of the institution at large.

Campus housing policy must rest on the best currently available medical information about HIV infection and AIDS. Of special note are the following facts:

1. HIV is not transmitted by any form of casual contact. No evidence supports the existence of any risk of transmission to household or residential contacts. **There is no justification for excluding students with AIDS, an AIDS-related illness, or positive tests for antibody to HIV from residential housing in order to protect others from casual transmission. On the other hand, immuno-compromised students, whether they have an AIDS-related disorder or another illness, may require special housing arrangements for their own protection from casually transmissible organisms.**

2. HIV is transmitted by intimate sexual contact and exposure to contaminated blood, usually through the sharing of needles for injecting illicit drugs. **Protection against these exposures requires education of all students and employees; it is not accomplished by excluding those with AIDS, an AIDS-related illness, or a positive test for antibody to HIV from residence halls.**

3. **AIDS, an AIDS-related illness, and a positive test for antibody to HIV are conditions present in individuals, not in buildings.** Whether individuals who are infected with HIV transmit the virus is not determined by where they live or whether they live together.

The most important feature of any AIDS-related housing policy is a good educational program. Most students with HIV infection will not be identified or recognized as such. Many infected individuals do not realize that they are infected, and many who are aware of their infection will choose not to disclose it to college and university officials. In developing housing policy, it is important to understand that *identified* students with HIV infection will probably represent a minority of those infected. Housing policies that are unnecessarily restrictive or that weaken the security of confidential information will decrease students' willingness to disclose their HIV infection or seek appropriate services.

Since HIV is transmitted only by certain intimate behaviors and since many infected students will not be identified, the most appropriate and effective means of limiting the spread of HIV infection will be through widespread educational programs.

GUIDELINES FOR HOUSING AND RESIDENCE LIFE PROGRAMS

The following recommendations and guidelines recognize certain specific features of the close cooperation necessary among various units of the institution to guarantee an appropriate and consistent response to AIDS-related housing issues.

1. **Identify a campus task force to serve the community as a working group to respond to AIDS-related concerns** . . . It might appropriately include directors or representatives of the health service, counseling center, food services, housing, and the personnel office, among others. The task force should determine the impact of applicable federal and state laws or judicial decisions before recommending policies.

2. **For both legal and ethical reasons and in light of the medical evidence, ACHA strongly discourages the adoption of policies that exclude or remove persons having AIDS, an AIDS-related illness, or a positive test for antibody to HIV from campus housing.** Since students with AIDS or an AIDS-related illness are regarded as "handicapped" by their medical condition, institutional officers must consider the applicability of the Rehabilitation Act of 1973, which prohibits discrimination against "qualified handicapped individual(s)" in programs or activities conducted with federal assistance.

3. **Identify principal individuals delegated the responsibility of coordinating AIDS education among faculty, staff, and students.** These individuals should stay aware of new information about HIV infection and AIDS, be informed about policies at comparable institutions, and attempt to foster an objective and informed attitude about HIV infection and AIDS in the institution. Housing and residence life officers must work closely with these people to provide good educational programming for residence hall staff and residents, as well as for maintenance, clerical, and other housing support staff. Residence hall staff should be educated prior to the arrival of students each fall. A comprehensive educational program does not stop after the initial presentations are over; periodic updates and reviews, with an oppor-

tunity for discussion, will promote effectiveness. Residence life programs provide an ideal setting for implementing peer education about HIV infection and AIDS . . .

4. **All housing and residence life staff should be able to identify campus and community resources for referrals for counseling, HIV antibody testing and medical evaluation, and education.**

5. **Housing and residence life staff should understand and observe the legal requirements and obligations concerning confidentiality of information.** Only a careful explanation of the importance of *unwavering adherence* to these requirements and a willingness to take strong measures against those who violate them will enable campus officials to reassure students that individual privacy and medical confidentiality are respected and protected by institutional personnel. The housing and residence life programs should establish procedures to deal with rumors about students alleged to have AIDS, an AIDS-related illness, or a positive test for antibody to HIV, and should limit participation in rumor-spreading by institutional staff by all reasonable means . . .

6. **It is important to encourage students with AIDS, an AIDS-related illness, or a positive test for antibody to HIV to inform health officials of their condition to promote their best medical care.** The health service should make arrangements at the earliest possible time to inform immunocompromised students of outbreaks of highly contagious diseases that pose a particular danger to them (e.g., chicken pox, measles) in order to reduce their chance of exposure. Effective implementation of such a plan depends upon close cooperation among the housing office, the residence life program, and the health service staff. Only information essential to guarantee the protection of the students involved must be transmitted.

7. **A single campus official should be designated to respond to inquiries from parents about a known or suspected student who is on campus and who has AIDS, or AIDS-related illness, or a positive test for antibody to HIV.** Housing and residence life officers should be prepared to direct such inquiries to this official . . .

8. **Under no circumstances should housing officials allow concern or suspicion about the health, sexual orientation, or sexual behavior of a student on the part of other students or employees to result in action taken against the suspected student.** Neither policy nor practice should allow such a student to be forced to be tested for antibody to HIV, relocated, isolated, ostracized, or excluded from campus housing. Both policy and practice should include strong and effective responses to harassment of any kind toward students.

RECOMMENDATIONS FOR A CAMPUS HOUSING POLICY

Recognizing that institutional circumstances vary, the American College Health Association suggests that campus officials consider the following options to protect healthy students; those with AIDS, an AIDS-related illness, or a positive test for antibody to HIV; and the institution itself.

1. To protect the student with AIDS, an AIDS-related illness, or a positive test for antibody to HIV.

a. **Communicable disease alert.** Develop a mechanism (1) to inform immunocompromised students about highly contagious diseases that may be of particular danger to them and (2) to identify protective measures to reduce such risk after consultation with health officials. Be certain that no unnecessary compromise of confidential information occurs in the appropriate performance of this function. Information can be passed along to all students through networks, such as resident assistants, without the need to know which students are infected with HIV. Such "general" advisories are important because many infected students are not recognized.

In addition, though a variety of educational strategies, encourage persons with AIDS, an AIDS-related illness, or a positive test for antibody to HIV to inform a campus health care provider about their condition, with the understanding that such information will be regarded as protected, confidential medical information. Only the success of this effort will allow the effective dissemination of a communicable disease alert. Health care providers can then notify immunocompromised students of the presence of and recommendations against contagious diseases.

b. **Cooperation and support.** Encourage the student with AIDS, an AIDS-related illness, or a positive test for antibody to HIV to discuss his or her situation with certain other campus officials, such as a counselor, chaplain, dean in the residence life program, or therapist, on a confidential basis in order that potential difficulties can be anticipated. It is important that all such students have someone they can turn to for advice, support, and understanding. Colleges and universities may wish to publish a list of campus officials who have been properly prepared to effectively handle the AIDS-related concerns of students.

c. **Restriction of information.** When a student assigned to a residence hall is known to have a positive test for antibody to HIV, a diagnosis of an AIDS-related illness, or AIDS, special sensitivities and care are required. As with any medical condition, confidentiality of the student's health status must be assured, not only on behalf of the student's rights but for overall confidence in the confidentiality of students' medical records.

111

In particular, housing or residential life staff who are aware that an HIV infected student has chosen or been assigned to share a room or an apartment with another student should anticipate many concerns. A highly competent counselor, health care professional, or administrator who is already aware of the student's HIV infection can offer assistance in discussing options and implications with respect to the student's roommate. **Under no circumstances should any college official violate the privacy of a student with HIV infection in order to inform other parties who might then counsel the student.** Only an official to whom the student has disclosed the fact of HIV infection or authorized (in writing) to be given that information can initiate discussions with the student.

The student with HIV infection may want to consider openly discussing his or her medical condition with the roommate. Such a discussion is not a requirement, and no student should be forced to disclose confidential medical information to a roommate. If the relationship between roommates is a strong one, though, the student with HIV infection may gain strength, understanding, and assistance from the roommate. This is especially important for a student infected with HIV who is asymptomatic initially but

---

Any discussion about relocating a student should involve careful consideration of the consequences of such a move.

---

manifests signs and symptoms of HIV infection that become obvious to the roommate later in the year.

The unpredictable response by a student who was unaware of the roommate's HIV status must be considered. Roommates who discover later that they have been living with a student with HIV infection may feel deceived and angry and may involve their parents in their response. Students with HIV infection should be aware of this possibility but also should know that the institution will generally defend their right to confidentiality of information. Should the student with HIV infection wish to keep the medical condition a private matter, not to be discussed with any others, the institution's representative should honor this request and protect the student's right to privacy. The institution should provide resources for concerned roommates as well, for education, counseling, and reassurance.

Each situation needs to be addressed on a case-by-case basis with consideration given to the HIV infected student, the rights of the roommate, and the potential impact upon the institution itself. By and large, roommates are protected by educational programs and their own behavior choices. It is difficult to see why a roommate would have a "right" or "need" to know that a student was infected with HIV.

d. **Relocation.** Depending on the individual medical and social circumstances involved, it may be appropriate to provide special housing arrangements for students with AIDS or an AIDS-related illness. Those who are immunocompromised should be offered the option of separate (single) living quarters or a room to accommodate a caretaker. Any discussion about relocating a student should involve careful consideration of the consequences of such a move—e.g., attention that may be drawn to the student's special circumstances by virtue of the relocation; ridicule, harassment, or other abuse; the student's own feelings of being ostracized and excluded. Thus, such a relocation should be accomplished only after thorough discussion with the student involved and only with his or her informed consent.

e. **Medical monitoring.** Encourage the affected student to participate in a program of regular medical follow-up and monitoring of his or her condition by health care personnel familiar with AIDS-related problems.

2. **To protect other students and employees from transmission of HIV by a student with AIDS, an AIDS-related illness, or a positive test for antibody to HIV.**

a. **Education of the affected student.** Through the health care provider, assess the affected student's knowledge about the transmission of HIV and the ways and means of preventing it. Provide, or arrange for, detailed education of the affected student and emphasize the need to behave responsibly in order to limit the risk of infecting others.

b. **Education of other students and staff.** Provide an effective and ongoing AIDS education program for all students and employees of the institution. Educational programs should reach housing and residence life employees prior to the arrival of students in the fall. Students living in campus housing should be educated shortly after their arrival.

3. **To protect the institution from adverse publicity, loss of students, or other consequences because of knowledge or rumor of students with AIDS, an AIDS-related illness, or a positive test for antibody to HIV.**

a. **Early identification, medical care, and education.** Encourage students with AIDS, an AIDS-related illness, or a positive test for antibody to HIV to inform a campus health care provider about their condition. Provide, or arrange for, competent and frequent medical follow-up and for detailed education of the affected student(s) regarding the transmission of HIV and the steps necessary to prevent it. Provide effective and ongoing educational programs for all other students and for institutional employees so they will be aware of preventive behaviors.

b. **Policies and procedures.** Develop policies and procedures for dealing with students with AIDS, an AIDS-related illness, or a positive test for antibody to HIV. Guarantee that such policies and procedures conform with applicable federal and state law. Be certain that they are well understood and consistently applied throughout the institution . . .

c. **Confidentiality.** Guarantee that confidential medical information about students with AIDS, an AIDS-related illness, or a positive test for antibody to HIV is protected. The inadvertent or malicious "leaking" of such information can cause extremely painful consequences for the affected students and the institution. All who might potentially deal with confidential medical information should clearly understand these facts . . .

d. **Public relations.** Appoint a single official to respond to public inquiries. He or she should state the institution's policy forthrightly and clearly, but should absolutely refuse to provide any specific information about individual students or residence halls . . .

Appendix VI

Policy Considerations

Q— What policies should we institute for the disposal of classroom waste? Do we need to be concerned, for example, about bloody facial tissues or adhesive bandages that might be thrown away in classroom garbage cans?

A— Garbage cans should be lined with plastic bags which facilitate disposal of waste. There is little reason to be concerned with the occasional bloody piece of waste disposed of in the usual fashion, but school personnel should be informed that trash contaminated with blood and body fluid should be bagged for disposal. This is particularly important if a large amount of waste is involved, for example, large quantities of towels or kleenex used to stop a nosebleed. Disposable gloves and bleach solutions should be available in all areas.

Q— What procedures do custodial personnel need to follow?

A— All custodial workers, like all other employees and staff, should be educated about the risks of HIV infection because of contact with blood or body fluids, but it should be emphasized how remote the risk is. Gloves should be provided as well as appropriate disinfectants.

Q— What should we do if a student is exposed to blood from an individual known to be infected with HIV?

A— If the exposure is a surface exposure only, thorough cleaning with soap and water and an antibacterial solution should suffice. Unless the exposure involves broken skin, there is almost no risk of transmitting HIV infection. If exposure is parenteral, such as a needlestick or other blood to blood contact, referral to a physician trained to evaluate and follow up such exposure is necessary. At the present time, there is no prophylactic treatment which can prevent infection by HIV if a substantial exposure occurs. Most needlestick or other small parenteral exposures do not appear to transmit HIV infection, and care is generally limited to sequential testing to determine whether antibody develops, as well as instituting appropriate personal precautions, such as the use of condoms during sexual intercourse, until it can be determined with relative certainty that infection has not occurred (a period of one to two years).

Q— Is it permissible to require HIV testing as a part of a physical exam for scholarship football players?

A— Probably not. A general physical exam to determine present fitness is certainly appropriate, and this may reveal indications that the student is infected with HIV and symptomatic from his infection. If the effects are sufficient to render the student unfit to play football, he may be excluded, not on the basis of his infection but because of the physical infirmity HIV infection has produced. If the physical exam reveals some cause to suspect that HIV infection is present, it may be incumbent on the physician to order appropriate diagnostic tests to confirm or exclude this possibility, but the fact of HIV infection alone cannot be used as a basis for exclusion from team play or scholarship consideration if anti-discrimination laws apply. It is best not to adopt a policy of screening athletes for HIV infection.

Q— Suppose a student who is known to be infected with HIV is also known to be having unprotected intercourse with partners who are unaware of his infection. Assuming this is occurring in a residence hall, and assuming the student is resistant to suggestions that he modify his behavior, does the school have a duty to inform the partners of the student's HIV infection?

A— It is uncertain whether there is a duty to warn, but it appears that disclosure without consent of the student is very likely to be actionable as an invasion of privacy. In such a circumstance, the safest course of action is to report the student's activity to the public health authorities and allow them to handle the problem. If the student's actions are, independent of the fact of HIV infection, in violation of school or residence hall rules, independent grounds for dismissal or expulsion from the residence hall may exist and may be pursued, as long as the rules have historically been evenhandedly applied to all students. Situations such as these present the greatest risk to administrators who must address them; legal counsel should always be consulted because the most appropriate course of action may vary considerably depending on the facts of the particular situation.

Q— Do any special precautions need to be made for common laundry, toilet or eating facilities in residence halls.

A— Aside from general principles of hygiene, no.

Glossary

Discussion of AIDS requires some familiarity with medical terms. Below is a summary of the medical terms used in this monograph. The reader is cautioned that the definitions here are directed specifically toward the monograph discussion of HIV infection, and are not always general definition.

AIDS—Acquired immune deficiency syndrome, a viral disease caused by infection with HIV

Antibody—a blood protein produced by cells of the immune system in response to immunological stimulation, such as infection by virus. In many cases the production of antibody results in immunity against the agent which prompted production of the antibody. This does not seem to be so with antibody to HIV, which does not protect the host from ill effects of infection but does indicate that infection has occurred.

Antibody titre—the level of antibody present in the blood.

Asymptomatic—showing no symptoms of disease although infected. Also known as silent or latent infection.

ARC—AIDS-related complex, a symptomatic form of HIV infection which is clinically less severe than AIDS. ARC may evolve into AIDS.

CDC—Center(s) for Disease Control.

Communicable Disease—any disease which can be transmitted from one individiual to another; also known as infectious disease.

ELISA—a screening test used for determination of antibody to HIV. This test is used both to eliminate tainted blood from blood bank supplies and as the initial screening test to determine whether an individual is infected by HIV. Because it has a high possibility of false

117

positive results, it must be followed by another confirmatory test, usually the Western Blot, if confirmation of HIV infection is needed.

Intrauterine Transmission—infection of the infant while still in the womb.

Immunosuppressed—having an immune system which is not functioning properly; also called immune compromised.

Lymphocytes—white blood cells which are a primary part of the body's immune response. HIV infection causes a decrease in particular subsets of lymphocytes.

Opportunistic Infection—infection by an organism not usually causing human disease. Opportunistic infections are common whenever the immune system is not functioning properly and are very common in ARC and AIDS.

Parenteral Exposure—exposure to a substance by a penetrating route, such as needlestick or injection.

Seronegative—lacking antibody to HIV.

Seropositive—having antibody to HIV.

Venereal Disease—a communicable or infectious disease ordinarily transmitted by sexual contact.

Western Blot—a confirmatory test for the presence of HIV infection. A positive Western Blot means that the individual has definitely been infected by HIV.

Cases Cited

Acosta v. Carey, 365 So.2d 4 (La. App. 1978).

Berry v. Moench, 8 Utah 2d 191, 331 P.2d 814 (1958).
Bowers v. Harwicke, 106 S. Ct. 2841 (1986).
Brady v. Hopper, 570 F. Supp. 1333 (Dist. Colo. 1983).
Bratt v. IBM Corp., 392 Mass. 508, 467 N.E.2d 126 (Mass. 1984).

Campbell v. Talladega County Board of Education, 518 F. Supp. 47 (N.D. Ala. 1981).
Chrysler Outboard Corp. v. Dilhr, 14 FEP Cases 394 (Wisc. Cir. Ct. 1976).
Craig v. Boren, 429 U.S. 190 (1976).
Cronan v. New England Telephone, Civil Action No. 80332 (Sup. Ct. Aug. 16, 1986).
Cordero v. Coughlin, 607 F. Supp. (S.D.N.Y. 1984).

Derrick v. Ontario Community Hospital, 47 Cal. App. 3d 145, 120 Cal. Rptr. 566 (Cal. Ct. App. 1975).
District 27 Community School Board v. Board of Education of City of New York, 130 Misc. 2d 398, 502 N.Y.S.2d 325 (Sup. Ct. N.Y. 1986).
Dunn v. Blumstein, 405 U.S. 330 (1972).
Duvall v. Golden, 362 N.W.2d 275 (Mich. Ct. App. 1984).

E.E. Black Co. v. Marshall, 497 F. Supp. 1088 (D. Hawaii 1980).

Florida v. Dunn, 86-66 CF (Union County, Florida).

Gammil v. U.S., 727 F.2d 950 (10th Cir. 1984).

Graham v. Richardson, 403 U.S. 365 (1971).

Grove City College v. Bell, 465 U.S. 555 (1984).

Horne v. Patton, 291 Ala. 701, 287 So.2d 824 (1973).

Indiana v. Haines, Tippecanoe Super. Ct. No. 5-5585.

Jacobsen v. Massachusetts, 197 U.S. 11 (1905).

Jew Ho v. Williamson, 103 F. 10 (N.D.Cal. 1900).

Johnson by Johnson v. Ann Arbor Public Schools, 569 F. Supp. 1502 (E.D. Mich. 1983).

Kaiser v. Suburban Transportation System, 398 P.2d 14 (Wash. 1965).

Kirk v. Board of Health, 83 S.C. 372, 65 S.E. 387 (1909).

Korematsu v. United States, 323 U.S. 214 (1944).

Lipari v. Sears, Roebuck, 497 F. Supp. 185 (D. Neb. 1985).

MacDonald v. Clinger, 446 N.Y.S.2d 801 (N.Y. Sup. Ct. 1982).

Mikel v. Abrams, 541 F. Supp. 591 (W.D. Mo. 1982).

New York State Society of Surgeons v. Axelrod.

New York City Transit Authority v. Beazer, 440 U.S. 568 (1978).

Oyama v. California, 332 U.S. 633 (1948).

People v. Prairie Chicken, CRE-77357 (El Cajon, California).

People v. Richards, 85-1715FH (Flint, Michigan).

Poole v. South Plainfield Board of Education, 490 F. Supp. 948 (D.C. N.J. 1980).

Ray v. School District of DeSoto County, no. 87-88-CIV-FtM-17(c), slip. op. (M.D. Fla. August 5, 1987).

School Board of Nassau County v. Arline, 107 S. Ct. 1123 (1987).

Shuttleworth v. Broward County, 639 F. Supp. 654 (S.D. Fla. 1986); 639 F. Supp. 35 (S.D. Fla. 1986).

Simonsen v. Swenson. 104 Neb. 224, 117 N.W. 831 (1920).

State Association for Retarded Persons v. Carey, 466 F. Supp. 479 (E.D. N.Y. 1978); aff'd. 612 F.2d 644 (2d Cir. 1979).

State Division of Human Rights v. Xerox Corp., 65 N.Y.2d 213 (1985).

Tarasoff v. Board of Regents of the University of California, 131 Cal. Rep. 15, 17 Cal.3d 358, 551 P.2d 334 (1974).

Thompson v. County of Alameda, 27 Cal.3d 741, 167 Cal. Rptr. 70, 614 P.2d 728 (1980).

White v. Western School Corp., No. IP-85-1192-C (slip. op.) (1985).

Wong Wai v. Williamson, 103 F. 1 (N. D. Cal. 1900).

Wright v. Columbia University, 520 F. Supp. 789 (E. D. Pa. 1981).

Bibliography

Baker, The Teacher's Right to Know Versus the Student's Right to Privacy, 16 J, *Law and Education* 71 (1987).

Bodine, Opening the Schoolhouse Door for Children with AIDS, 13 *Bost. Coll. Env. Aff. L.R.* 583 (1986).

CDC, Immunization of children infected with human T-lymphotrophic virus type III/lymphadenopathy associated virus, 35 *MMWR* 595 (1986).

Cecere, Working With AIDS, 16 *Brief* 4, 11 (1987).

Constitutional Rights of AIDS Carriers, 99 *Harvard L.R.* 1275 (1986).

Coolfront Report, A Public Health Service Plan for Prevention and Control of AIDS and the AIDS virus, 101 *Public Health Reports* 347 (1986).

Curran (I), et. al., AIDS: Legal and Regulatory Policy, U.S. Department of Health and Human Services 330 (1986).

Curran (II), et. al., AIDS: Legal and Policy Implications of the Application of Traditional Disease Control Measures, 15 *Law Medicine and Health Care* 27, 28 (1986).

Fox, From TB to AIDS: Value Conflicts in Reporting Disease, 16 *Hastings Center Report* (Supp) 11 (1986).

Field and Sullivan, AIDS and the Criminal Law, 15 *Law Medicine and Health Care*, 46, 49 (1987).

Gostin, The Limits of Compulsion in Controlling AIDS, 16 *Hastings Center Report* (Supp.) 24 (1986).

Gostin et. al. The Case Against Compulsory Casefinding in Controlling AIDS: Testing , Screening and Reporting, 12 *American J. Law and Medicine* 7, 50 (1987).

Hermann, Liability Related to Diagnosis and Transmission of AIDS, 15 *Law, Medicine and Health Care* 36 (1987).

Kaplan and Kleinman, Serologic Tests for Infection with Human Immunodeficiency Virus, 17 *Laboratory Medicine* 690, 691 (1986).

Keeling, AIDS on the College Campus: *ACHA Special Report* 5 (1986).

Lamb, To Tell or Not To Tell: Physician Liability for Disclosure of Patient Information, 13 *Cumberland L.R.* 593 (1983).

Lipton, Blood Donor Sources and Liability Issues Related to the Acquired Immune Deficiency Syndrome, 7 *Journal of Legal Medicine* 131 (1986).

Merritt, The Constitutional Balance Between Health and Liberty, 16 *Hastings Center Report* (Supp) 2 (1986).

National Education Association, Guidelines for Dealing with AIDS in the Schools (1986).

Parmet, AIDS and the Limits of Discrimination Law, 15 *Law Medicine and Health Care* 61, 69 (1987).

Schilts, Randy, *And the Band Played On*, St. Martin's Press, Viking Penguin Books, copyright 1987 (1st printing).

Steinbach, J., AIDS on Campus: Emerging Issues for College and University Administrators, *American Council on Education* (1987).

Stone, The Tarasoff Decisions: Suing Psychotherapists to Safeguard Society, 91 *Harvard L.R.* 358 (1976).

U.S. Dept. of Health and Human Services, Current Status of State Law Regarding AIDS (August 1987).

Resources for Legal Information in Secondary and Higher Education

MONOGRAPHS

If you have found the information contained in this monograph to be helpful in your day-to-day operations or as a reference, it is quite likely that you may also be interested in other titles included in our *Higher Education Administration Series* of monographs. For a complete list of titles at the time of this printing, refer to the order blank on the next page.

PERIODICALS

The periodicals listed on the order form (next page), offer the reader a quarterly report on recent precedent setting higher court decisions covering a wide range of subjects in the area encompassed by each self-descriptive title. In addition, through the accumulated back issues—and in the "College" publications, a casebook—each of these publications are also excellent comprehensive references that can be of great help in day-to-day operations and long range planning.

The last title, *SYNTHESIS: Law and Policy in Higher Education*, published five times yearly, briefs its readers on key issues involving law and policy in higher education. *SYNTHESIS*, with its unique "one-on-one" format that devotes each issue entirely to one topic, is an excellent way for educators and administrators to refresh and update their understanding of key law and policy issues affecting their policy-making and day-to-day operations.

Pricing of the publications listed was correct at the time of publication of this monograph. If you want further information or current prices before shipment, please enter a "?" in the total column at the right of that item on the order blank on the reverse side.

Order Blank *(Orders will be shipped & billed at current prices)*

| Qty. | CAP # | Item | Price | Total |

MONOGRAPHS

____ 04 Administering College and University Housing.......$12.95*   _____

____ 05 The Dismissal of Students with Mental Disorders.....$12.95*   _____

____ 06 A Practical Guide to Legal Issues Affecting
         College Teachers................................$6.95†   _____

____ 07 Computers in Education: Legal Liabilities and
         Ethical Issues Concerning Their Use and Misuse.....$12.95*   _____

____ 08 Faculty / Staff Nonrenewal and Dismissal for Cause
         in Institutions of Higher Education.................$12.95*   _____

____ 09 Guide to Successful Searches for College Personnel...$12.95*   _____

____ 10 Academic Integrity and Student Development ....$12.95*   _____

____ 12 Crime and Campus Police:
         A Handbook for Police Officers & Administrators...$12.95*   _____

____ 13 Alcohol on Campus: A Compendium of the Law
         and a Guide to Campus Policy....................$39.95   _____

____ 14 The Educators Guide to AIDS:
         Law, Medicine and Policy........................$12.95*   _____

PERIODICALS

____ 01 The College Student and the Courts
         Includes casebook, all back issues and four
         quarterly updating supplements..................$108.50   _____

____ 02 The College Administrator and the Courts
         Includes casebook, all back issues and four
         quarterly updating supplements..................$108.50   _____

____ 03 The Schools and the Courts
         Includes over 600 pages of back issues and four
         updating reports................................$95.50   _____

____ 11 Synthesis: Law and Policy in Higher Education
         Five issues per academic year ....$59.50   _____

* *Ten or more copies @ $9.95*
† *Ten or more copies @ $4.95*   *N.C. residents add sales tax*   _____
‡ *We will add shipping charges to invoice*
  if order is not prepaid.   TOTAL‡   _____

Bill to:..........................   *Ship to:*..........................

....

....

Authorized by:.....................   ....
(Print Name)   Signature

Address Orders to:

College Administration Publications, Inc., Dept. CP
P.O. Box 8492, Asheville, NC 28814   —   *or phone (704) 252-0883*

☐ *For further information or current prices on above titles please indicate with check
   here and "?" in the quantity column.*